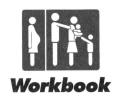

Workbook

American Red Cross Healthy Pregnancy, Healthy Baby

This program is solely educational and is not intended to be a substitute for medical advice or care. Participants who have specific concerns and questions about their own conditions should contact their personal health care provider.

ISBN: 0-86536-196-7

Acknowledgments

This course and textbook were developed and produced by the members of the development team at American Red Cross national headquarters. The development team researched, wrote, designed, and tested the course. Team members include Donna M. Feeley, M.P.H., project director; Julie Huff, B.S.N., project analyst; and Barbara J. Monfort, M.P.A., project analyst.

Many individuals contributed their expertise and support in creative and technical ways. The course could not have been developed without the assistance of Thomas Edwards and Joan Timberlake for editing, Jane Moore for desktop publishing, and Sheila O. Powell and Betty Butler for administrative support.

The following national headquarters Health and Safety volunteers and paid staff provided review and assistance: Robert F. Burnside, director, Health and Safety; Frank Carroll, manager, Development; Ann P. Dioda, associate, Operations; Cynthia Vlasich, R.N., manager, External Relations; Dennis L. Zaenger, M.P.H., associate; Stephen Silverman, Ed.D., volunteer consultant; and Rose Yuhos, R.N., chairman, National Nursing Advisory Committee.

Special thanks and appreciation go to Keith Dana of Design Consultants for the cover art and his illustrations.

Guidance and technical assistance were also provided by members of the American Red Cross Healthy Pregnancy, Healthy Baby Advisory Committee. Gratitude is extended to these individuals who shared their organizations' valuable resources, as well as their own time and expertise in reviewing these materials:

Deborah M. Bash, C.N.M., M.S.N.
Acting Director, Nurse Midwifery Program
Georgetown University School of Nursing
Graduate Program
Washington, D.C.

Gwendolyn Bradford, R.N., M.S.
Assistant Professor
Howard University School of Nursing
Washington, D.C.

Pamela Frable, N.D., R.N.*
Chairperson
Healthy Pregnancy, Healthy Baby Advisory Committee
Director, Health Services
American Red Cross
Tarrant County Chapter
Ft. Worth, Texas

*Special thanks go to these committee members who helped coordinate and implement the pilot test.

Ron Frick
Director, Safety & Health
American Red Cross
Greater New York Chapter
New York, New York

Anna J. Jenkins, B.S.N.*
Parent Education Coordinator
Deaconess Medical Center
Spokane, Washington

Lt. Comdr. Donna Kahn, C.P.N.P., M.S.N.
Pediatrics Nurse Practitioner
Naval Medical Clinic
Annapolis, Maryland

Col. Elizabeth A. (Betty) MacDonald, M.S.N., R.N.C.
Consultant for Nursing Affairs
Office of the Surgeon General
U.S. Air Force
Washington, D.C.

Capt. June Mikkila, B.S.N., M.P.H.*
Chief Community Health Nurse
Preventive Medicine
Ft. Devens, Massachusetts

Ellen Neiman, B.S.N., M.S.
Lt. Col. (Ret.) U.S. Army
Tucson, Arizona

Col. Marie R. O'Neil, M.S.N.
Chief, Community Health Nursing
Brooke Army Medical Center
Ft. Sam Houston, Texas

Celeste R. Phillips, R.N., Ed.D.
Principal, Phillips and Fenwick
Scotts Valley, California

Barbara Scherek, R.N., B.S.*
Nursing Specialist, Health and Safety
American Red Cross
European Area Headquarters

The following individuals helped coordinate and implement the pilot test. These materials could not have been produced without their dedication and commitment:

Diane Benning, B.S.N.
Assistant Station Manager
American Red Cross
Sembach, Germany

Billie Moultrie, M.S.N.
Volunteer Chairperson
Nursing Committee
American Red Cross
Sembach, Germany

Acknowledgments

Carol Ireland, M.S.
Assistant Station Manager
American Red Cross
Stuttgart, Germany

Jacquelyn J. Duarte, B.S.N., M.P.A.
Nursing Chair
American Red Cross
Naples, Italy

Sammie K. Grier-Brooks
PFP Instructor
American Red Cross
Naples, Italy

Karen T. Woodward
Station Manager
American Red Cross
Naples, Italy

External technical review was provided by the following individuals. Grateful appreciation is also extended to them:

Mary Ann Braun, R.N.C., M.S.N., O.G.N.P.
Director of Practice and Legislation
Organization for Obstetric, Gynecologic, and
    Neonatal Nurses
Washington, D.C.

Denise M. Combs, R.N.C., A.C.C.E.
Volunteer Nursing Chairman
American Red Cross
Station Manager's Office
Ft. Riley, Kansas

Sarah Coulter Danner, M.S.N., C.N.M., C.P.N.P.
Director, Midwifery Program
MetroHealth Hospital for Women
Cleveland, Ohio

Carl Jones
Certified Childbirth Educator
Whitefield, New Hampshire

John H. Kennell, M.D.
Rainbow Babies and Children's Hospital
Cleveland, Ohio

Carole L. Kuhns, R.N., M.S.
Assistant Professor
Georgetown University School of Nursing
Washington, D.C.

Barbara L. Leighton, M.D.
Co-Director, Obstetric Anesthesia Department
Thomas Jefferson University Hospital
Philadelphia, Pennsylvania

Janet B. McCracken, M.Ed.
Early Childhood Education Consultant
Gettysburg, Pennsylvania

Deborah Davis Richards
Child Passenger Safety Specialist
Seattle, Washington

Leonard P. Rome, M.D.
Fellow, American Academy of Pediatrics
Shaker Heights, Ohio

Jerome J. Scherek, M.D.
Fellow
American College of Obstetricians and Gynecologists
Annandale, Minnesota

Bruce M. Shephard, M.D.
Clinical Associate Professor, Obstetrics & Gynecology
University of South Florida School of Medicine
Tampa, Florida

Linda Todd, M.P.H.
Perinatal Education Coordinator
Riverside Medical Center
Minneapolis, Minnesota

Betsy Vieth, M.P.H.
Deputy Director
Program to Strengthen Primary Care Health Centers
National Association of Community Health
    Centers, Inc.
Washington, D.C.

Contents

Introduction

Welcome to the American Red Cross Healthy Pregnancy, Healthy Baby course. This course was designed to give parents the knowledge they need to make informed choices during and after pregnancy. The focus is on healthy living and responsible decision making.

The American Red Cross Healthy Pregnancy, Healthy Baby course and this workbook consist of three modules: I. Healthy Pregnancy; II. Labor and Birth; and III. Family and Infant Care.

In Module I, you will learn about your changing body and feelings, how your body grows, nutrition and exercise, and how to enjoy pregnancy. In Module II, you will learn about labor and birth and their variations and ways to cope with pain and discomfort. In Module III, you will learn about what happens after birth, bringing your baby home, ways to prevent injury, and planning ahead.

Each chapter in the workbook begins with a short description of what the chapter covers. Some chapters contain think sheets for you to complete at home or in class. You will be discussing these think sheets in class. Some chapters have instructions on how to do physical and mental exercises. You will be practicing these exercises in class and at home. Time is allowed in the course for group discussion and for questions and answers. In addition, you will see several short videos about labor and birth and about caring for your newborn.

The workbook also contains appendixes that cover different aspects of childbirth and parenting, including a suggested reading list and a list of organizations that might be helpful to you. There is also a glossary that defines words that may be unfamiliar to you.

Enjoy your pregnancy!

Module I
Healthy Pregnancy

Congratulations! Maybe you've just found out that you are pregnant and are overwhelmed by many feelings. Maybe you've known for a long while and are wondering what you need to do. This module, "Healthy Pregnancy," discusses the changes that occur during pregnancy and how to care for yourself and your baby while you are pregnant. The module includes time for you to write down your thoughts and feelings and any questions you want to ask your health care provider. You will also practice exercises and skills in class to help you feel stronger and better during your pregnancy.

Chapter 1 covers how your body changes and how to cope with these changes. Chapter 2 discusses emotional and role changes during pregnancy and gives you and your partner some tools to help sort out some of these changes. In Chapter 3, you will learn how your baby grows and how best to take care of your baby inside the womb. Chapter 4 gives you an opportunity to think about and practice some skills (exercise, relaxation, and visualization) that will make your pregnancy more enjoyable.

1 *Your Changing Body*

In this chapter, you will learn—
- About your reproductive system during pregnancy.
- What to expect during each trimester.
- About weight gain during pregnancy.
- About the discomforts of pregnancy and how to cope with them.
- When to call your health care provider.
- How to take care of your body.
- Correct posture and conditioning exercises.

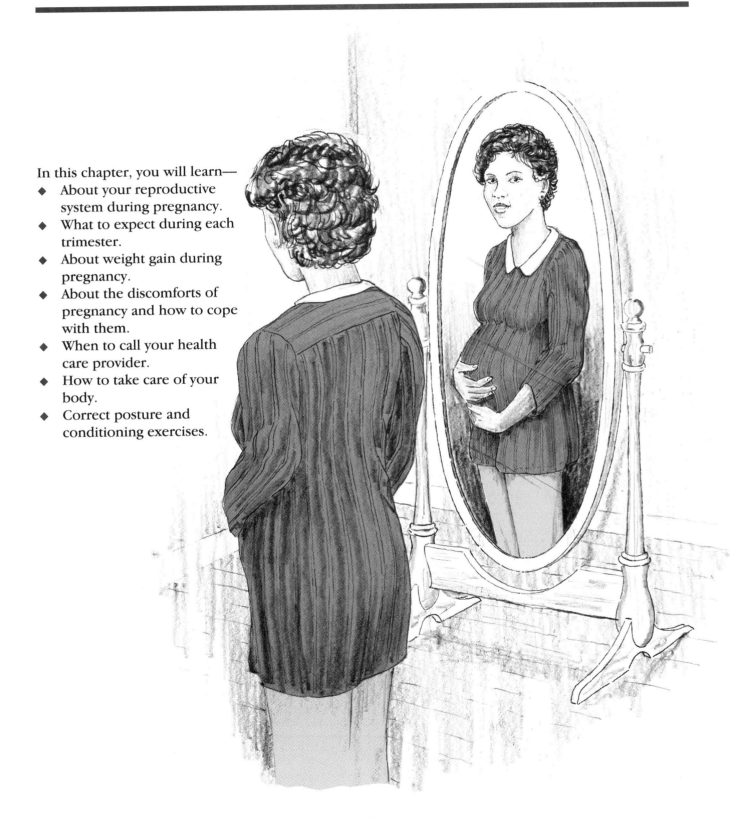

Your body may amaze you during pregnancy as it grows and changes to meet the demands of your baby. It can also be a source of concern and discomfort. Knowing what changes to expect, how to ease common discomforts, and how to care for your body during pregnancy will help you to feel good about yourself and your baby throughout pregnancy and after.

Basic Terms You Should Know

To understand what is happening in your body during pregnancy, you should understand the changes that are occurring. Following are some of the anatomical terms used to talk about pregnancy:

♦ **Uterus (womb)**—A hollow muscular organ. Normally the size and shape of a pear, it expands enough to hold a baby inside. There are three parts of the uterus: the fundus, which is the upper part; the body, or middle part; and the cervix, which is the lower part. The cervix extends into the vagina about 1-1/2 inches and has a small passageway that is normally closed tight. It opens during labor for the birth of the baby. During labor, the uterus contracts. Contractions, called Braxton Hicks contractions, occur throughout pregnancy. They are usually short and painless, but if you experience many of them, call your health care provider.

♦ **Vagina**—A muscular passage that connects the bottom of the uterus with the outside of the body.

♦ **Amniotic sac**—A fluid-filled bag composed of two separate thin layers. The sac holds amniotic fluid, the placenta, the umbilical cord, and the baby. The amniotic sac is sometimes called the "bag of waters" or the "membranes."

♦ **Amniotic fluid**—The fluid in which the baby floats inside the amniotic sac.

♦ **Placenta**—A spongy structure attached to the inside of the uterus during pregnancy, through which the baby receives nourishment and oxygen.

♦ **Umbilical cord**—A cord that attaches the baby to the placenta, through which nourishment and oxygen travel to the baby.

♦ **Round ligaments**—Ligaments that attach the uterus to the abdominal wall in the front of the body.

♦ **Pelvis**—The bony structure of the body through which the baby must pass. It consists of the pubic bone in front, the hip bones on the sides, and the end of the spine (the coccyx) in the back of the body.

♦ **Perineum**—The area between the vagina and the anus.

♦ **Pelvic floor**—Muscle layers at the bottom of the pelvis that support the uterus and the bladder.

The growing pregnancy (the uterus with the baby inside, the placenta, and the amniotic sac) results in changes in much of a woman's body. The stomach, intestines, and rectum may be crowded, the bladder compressed, and the backbone (sacrum) pushed outward in an exaggerated curve. These changes may cause various discomforts, but are not of major concern.

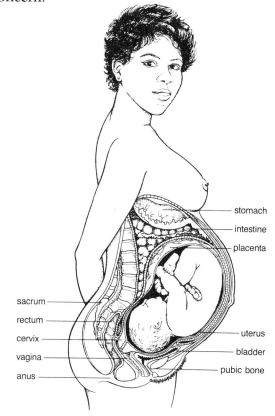

sacrum

rectum

cervix

vagina

anus

stomach

intestine

placenta

uterus

bladder

pubic bone

Trimester by Trimester

Pregnancy is divided into three three-month periods called trimesters. Listed below are some of the physical changes and feelings that women experience during each trimester. Some pregnant women experience only a few of these changes and feelings, while others may experience many or all.

First Trimester	Second Trimester	Third Trimester
No menstrual period	Quickening (beginning to feel the baby move)	Weight gain
Excitement	Weight gain	Desire for the baby to be born
Mixed emotions	Increased energy	Anxiety
Food cravings	Increased sexual desire	Mixed emotions
Frequent urination	Skin changes	Shortness of breath
Sensitive breasts	Mixed emotions	Backache
Nausea and vomiting	Heartburn	Fatigue
Fatigue	Excess gas	Bladder pressure
	Constipation	Swelling of the feet
	Round ligament pain	Insomnia
	Low back pain	Hemorrhoids
	Leg cramps	Varicose veins
	Hemorrhoids	
	Increased vaginal discharge	

Questions About Weight Gain

How much weight should I gain during my pregnancy?
Between 24 and 34 pounds.

How much weight should I gain each week?
Usually you will gain one to three pounds in the first trimester, then three-quarters to one pound a week through the rest of your pregnancy. If you gain or lose more than two pounds in a week, consult your health care provider. The chart below shows where the weight you gain during pregnancy actually goes.

What if I'm overweight already, can I diet?
No, you should not diet during pregnancy. Consult your health care provider concerning any changes you may want to make in your diet.

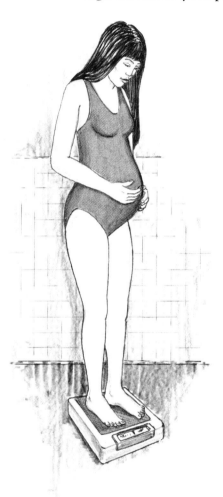

Estimated Weight Gain	*Where the Weight Goes*
4–8 pounds	Maternal stores (mother's fat, protein, other nutrients)
3–4 pounds	Increased fluid volume
3–4 pounds	Increased blood volume
2–3 pounds	Breast enlargement
2–3 pounds	Uterus
7–8 pounds	Baby
2 pounds	Amniotic fluid
1–2 pounds	Placenta
24–34 pounds	Total Estimated Weight Gain

My Pregnancy Record

Use this think sheet to record how you are feeling physically at this point in your pregnancy. Write down any actions you have taken to feel better or to relieve discomfort. Also list any questions regarding body changes that you want to ask your health care provider.

How I'm feeling physically

_____

_____

_____

_____

Actions taken

_____

_____

_____

_____

Questions for my health care provider

_____

_____

_____

_____

For fathers: Sometimes an expectant father feels discomforts or symptoms similar to the mother's. Have you felt any of these?

_____

_____

_____

_____

Discomforts of Pregnancy

A woman's body responds in many ways to pregnancy. Sometimes these responses result in physical discomfort for the pregnant woman. The chart below lists some of the discomforts and what causes them. It also shows ways you can help relieve the discomforts that may occur during pregnancy.

Discomfort	Cause	How to Help Yourself
Frequent Urination/ Leakage	Increased pressure of the uterus on your bladder during the first trimester. Baby putting pressure on your bladder in late pregnancy.	Drink less fluid before going to bed. Do Kegel exercises (see page 20).
Nausea and Vomiting	May result from changes in hormones.	Eat small, frequent meals. Before getting up, or for a snack if your stomach is upset, eat dry crackers or toast. Avoid strong-smelling, spicy, and greasy foods.
Fatigue	In the first trimester, due to hormonal changes. In the third trimester, due to increased weight and the size of the uterus.	Get extra rest. Drink more fluids during the day rather than in the evening if getting up to go to the bathroom becomes a problem. Limited amounts of exercise during the day may help.
Heartburn	Slowed digestion. Hormones cause slowed digestion and relax the valve between the stomach and esophagus.	Avoid fried and spicy foods. Also avoid drinking large amounts of fluids with meals. Sometimes drinking milk or eating ice cream helps.
Excess Gas	Slowed digestion due to changes in hormones.	Avoid fatty foods. Chew your food thoroughly.
Constipation	Slowed digestion due to changes in hormones. Sometimes a reaction to iron supplements.	Drink more fluids, especially water, and eat more fruits and roughage. (Include bran in your diet.) Get regular exercise. Try to establish regular bowel habits. Do not use laxatives or enemas.

Discomfort	Cause	How to Help Yourself
Round Ligament Pain (sharp pains along the sides of the abdomen)	Stretching and pressure from the uterus on round ligaments.	Support your abdomen with pillows when lying down. When getting up from a lying position, roll onto your side and push to a sitting position to decrease strain.
Low Back Pain	Enlarging uterus changes your center of gravity so you tend to tilt your pelvis forward, straining your back muscles.	Maintain good posture (see page 13). Keep your abdomen pulled in and your buttocks tight. Avoid straining from bending over. Always lift with your legs, rather than bending to lift. Wear low-heel shoes. Practice hands-and-knees pelvic tilt exercise (see page 17).
Leg Cramps	Increased pressure of the uterus on the nerves and veins that go to the legs.	Pull up your toes with your hands or push your heel against the floor or wall.
Hemorrhoids	Enlarging uterus presses on veins, slows blood flow, and causes veins to enlarge. Constipation may make this problem worse.	Eat more fruits, vegetables, whole grains, and bran cereals. Drink more water. Soak in a warm bath. Witch hazel reduces swelling. Get moderate exercise. Avoid standing for long periods. Kegel exercises (see page 20) increase blood flow to the area. Elevate your buttocks on pillows.
Shortness of Breath	Breathing becomes more rapid to meet your body's need for more oxygen. This is normal. Uterus pushes up on your diaphragm, giving you a feeling of less room to breathe. Your lungs are compressed by about one inch.	Relax and try breathing more deeply and at a slow pace. Stand or sit erect. Raise your arms over your head to give your lungs more space.

Discomfort	Cause	How to Help Yourself
Swelling of the Feet	Decreased blood flow from the legs due to pressure of the uterus on the veins of the legs.	Avoid tight clothing around your legs, such as knee-high stockings. Avoid sitting or standing for long periods. Rest with your legs elevated.
Varicose Veins	Hormones cause the veins to relax and expand.	Avoid knee-high stockings that are tight around the knees or calves. Avoid standing for long periods. Avoid crossing your legs at the knee. Rest often with your legs elevated. You may need to wear support hose. If you do, put the support hose on before getting out of bed in the morning.

For Fathers

Don't be surprised if you start to experience symptoms during your partner's pregnancy, such as nausea, food cravings, back pain, weight gain, or irritability. These feelings, which are very common among fathers-to-be, are known as the "couvade syndrome." Although the cause is not known, some believe that these symptoms occur because the father is trying to "feel and share" the pregnancy. It is also thought that these symptoms occur as a signal for you and your partner to pay attention to your feelings during the pregnancy.

Even if you don't experience any of these symptoms, don't worry. Many fathers can be sensitive and understanding about what their partner is going through without feeling any of these symptoms. Just know that, by sharing the pregnancy experience more fully, you and your partner will become closer and the pregnancy can be more enjoyable.

When to Call Your Health Care Provider

Warning Signs During Pregnancy

There are some discomforts or symptoms that may indicate a serious problem. If you experience any of the symptoms below call your health care provider:

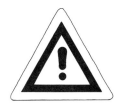

- Bleeding from your vagina.
- Persistent nausea or vomiting for longer than 24 hours (you can't keep anything down).
- Pain or burning when urinating.
- Fever and chills.
- Gush or trickle of water from your vagina.
- No activity of the baby for more than 12 hours (in the third trimester).
- Severe pain in your abdomen.
- Severe, persistent headache.
- Sudden swelling of your face, hands, feet, or ankles.
- Sudden, unexplained weight gain (more than two pounds in one week).
- Blurred vision or spots before your eyes.

Possible Signs of Premature Labor

Some of the signs that you are in premature labor are—

- Contractions that occur every 10 minutes or more often (five or more contractions in one hour).
- Menstrual-like cramps in your lower abdomen, which may come and go or be constant.
- Dull backache felt below your waistline, which may come and go or be constant.
- Pressure in your pelvis (feels like the baby is pushing down).
- Abdominal cramping, with or without diarrhea.
- Spotting or bleeding from your vagina.
- Watery discharge from your vagina.

IF ANY OF THESE SIGNS OCCUR, CALL YOUR HEALTH CARE PROVIDER IMMEDIATELY.

Questions About Body Care

Can I take a tub bath during pregnancy?
Showers or tub baths are fine during pregnancy. As you become bulkier, the difficulties and risks of getting in and out of the tub increase, so be careful. Once your bag of waters has broken, take only showers. Baths should be warm, not hot, since there is some evidence that extremely hot water harms the baby. Hot tubs and saunas should not be used during pregnancy.

Can I douche during pregnancy?
You should not douche because douching increases the risk of infection during pregnancy. It is not necessary to douche, even when you are not pregnant.

I'm planning to breastfeed. Is there anything I need to do to prepare my breasts?
Use only water when bathing your breasts and nipples because soap is drying. Massaging your breasts and nipples during the last two months of pregnancy may help condition and prepare them for breastfeeding. If you are at risk for premature labor, talk over breast preparation with your health care provider.

How much rest and sleep do I need during pregnancy?
Mothers should listen to their bodies. Rest when you need to. Lie down and put your feet up at least once during the day. Try to get at least eight hours of sleep a night. You may need more.

How do I stay comfortable?
If you stand most of the time, take a break, put up your feet and rest. If you sit most of the time, get up and move around every two to three hours to increase your circulation. Regular, mild exercise will help you sleep better at night. Use pillows to make yourself comfortable whenever you are lying down. Maintain good posture when you are standing or sitting.

Do I have to take special care of my teeth and gums during pregnancy?
If possible, take care of any dental problems before you become pregnant. However, if you have a toothache, contact a dentist because it could become serious if neglected. X rays should be avoided during pregnancy.

During pregnancy your gums may become puffy and bleed more easily because of hormonal changes. Therefore, it is important to brush and floss your teeth every day.

Posture

Following are some tips on maintaining good posture during pregnancy. Good posture is especially important during pregnancy. Your enlarging abdomen causes a shift in your center of gravity. Often you try to compensate by arching your back and sticking out your buttocks, causing extra strain on your back. In addition, the weight of your breasts may cause your shoulders to slump forward. Learning to be aware of your posture helps to make you more comfortable throughout your pregnancy. See *Figures 1, 2,* and *3* for appropriate posture positions.

Standing

Your neck should be straight. Lift your shoulders up and back; do not slouch forward. Make sure you are not leaning too far back. Tighten your stomach muscles, tucking your buttocks under and forward. Your knees should be relaxed and your weight should be distributed so that it is equal on both feet *(Fig. 1)*.

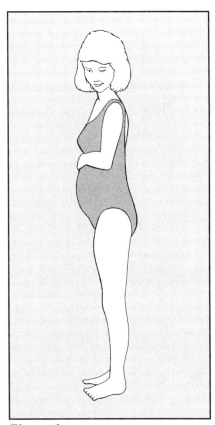

Figure 1
Standing

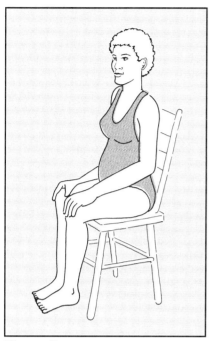

Figure 2
Sitting

Sitting

Your chair seat should support the length of your thigh. The height of the chair should allow your knees to be slightly elevated. Keep your legs slightly apart and not crossed. Keep your feet flat and parallel on the floor. Whenever possible, elevate your feet to increase circulation. If you sit at a desk for a long time, rest your head on your hands to relieve tension in your neck and shoulders *(Fig. 2).*

Lying Down

After the fourth month of pregnancy, you should lie on your side, preferably your left side. In this position, the weight of your uterus is not pressing on the major blood vessels of your body, and both you and the baby will get more blood flow. Experiment with pillows: try one or two pillows lengthwise between your legs to support the joints and a pillow under your head to support your head and upper arm. You may wish to put a small pillow under your abdomen *(Fig. 3).*

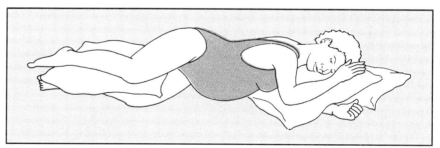

Figure 3
Lying down

Bending
Bend from your knees. When you are bending, your legs should be firmly planted in a comfortably wide stance to provide a broad base of support *(Fig. 4)*.

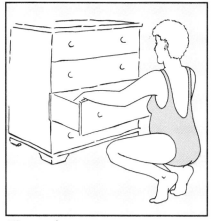

Figure 4
Bending

Lifting and Carrying
Use your thigh muscles to lift, rather than your back. Carry loads as close to your body as possible *(Fig. 5)*. Avoid twisting motions.

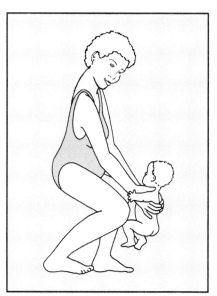

Figure 5
Lifting and carrying

Conditioning Exercises

Following are some conditioning exercises that you can do. Some of them, such as the pelvic tilt and the shoulder and upper-back exercises, help relieve aches and pains. Others, such as the tailor-sit and the Kegel exercises, condition muscles that are needed in childbirth itself.

Pelvic Tilt

The pelvic tilt is good for relieving back strain and strengthening abdominal muscles, as well as for reminding you to correct your posture during pregnancy. It can be done in many different positions. The easiest way to learn the pelvic tilt is to practice it while lying on your back. Practice in this position for only 10 to 15 minutes at a time. Once you know how to do the pelvic tilt, you can practice it in other positions. Try to do this exercise several times a day and whenever your back is aching. Following are instructions on how to do the pelvic tilt in various positions.

Lying on Your Back

Lie on your back with your feet flat on the floor, about hip distance apart. Your knees are bent. Put one hand under the small of your back and flatten your lower back onto the floor while you breathe in. As you breathe out, tighten your abdominal muscles and, at the same time, tighten the muscles in your buttocks *(Fig. 6).* Then relax. Repeat several times.

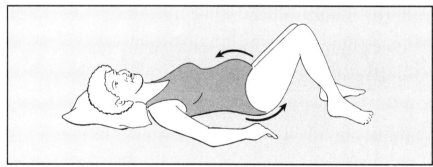

Figure 6
Pelvic Tilt
Lying on your back

Standing

Place one hand on your stomach and the other hand under your buttocks. Tighten your abdominal and buttock muscles at the same time. Tilt your hips forward *(Fig. 7)*. Relax your stomach muscles and release your hips. Repeat several times.

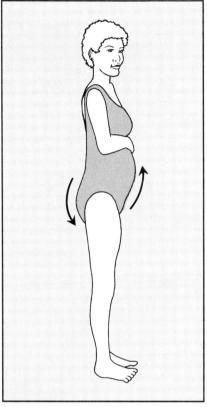

Figure 7
Pelvic Tilt
Standing

On Hands and Knees

When you are near the end of your pregnancy, this is a good position for doing the pelvic tilt. It gets the weight of the baby off of your back and provides some relief from back pain. While on your hands and knees, tilt your hips forward *(Fig. 8a)*. Then relax *(Fig. 8b)*. When you relax be sure that you do not let your spine sag or arch; just return to a position in which your back is flat.

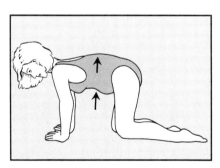

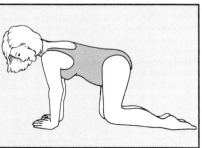

Figure 8a and b
Pelvic Tilt
On hands and knees

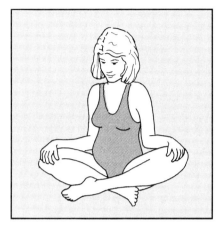

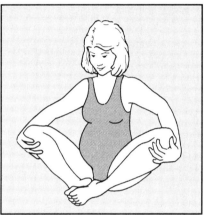

Figure 9a and b
Tailor-sitting

Tailor-sitting

Tailor-sitting helps to lengthen the muscles and ligaments of the inner thighs to prepare for birth. You may use the tailor-sit *(Fig. 9a)* any time—while talking on the telephone, watching television, etc. For an extra stretch, put your hands under your knees and push very gently against the hands *(Fig. 9b)*. If you have any pain, stop immediately. Change position after 10 minutes to promote good circulation. Do not put any downward pressure on your knees.

Shoulder and Upper-back Exercises

Because of changes in your center of gravity during pregnancy, you may tend to slump forward, resulting in upper-back pain. Here are two exercises to relieve upper-back pain and to remind you to keep your shoulders back:

Place your fingers on your shoulders and make backward circles with your shoulders and elbows *(Fig. 10)*.

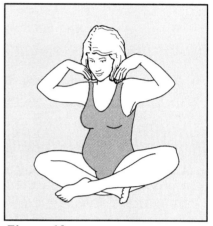

Figure 10
Shoulder

Stretch both of your arms over your head and reach first with the right arm, then with the left *(Fig. 11)*. Continue alternating upward arm reaches—right arm, then left arm—10 times. This relieves tightness in the shoulders and upper back and makes you feel as if you have more room to breathe.

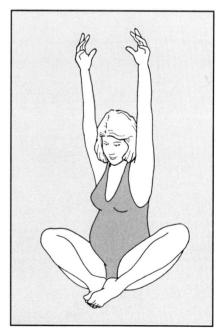

Figure 11
Upper back

Kegel Exercises (exercising the pelvic floor)

You should do Kegel exercises every day throughout your life. The muscles that form the floor of the pelvis support all the organs inside your body. They keep the bladder and the uterus in the proper position. Keeping these muscles strong aids in control of the bladder and enhances sexual pleasure for both partners.

Once you know how to do the Kegel exercises, you can do them any place, any time. They should be done at least 50 times a day but not all at once. This is how you practice:

◆ Tighten the muscles around the vagina and anus. (You may want to try this first by sitting on the toilet and practicing stopping and starting the flow of urine. Those are the same muscles you will use for this exercise.)

◆ Pull upward and inward as firmly as you can, and hold for three to five seconds.

◆ Relax. Then tighten these muscles slightly.

◆ Toward the end of pregnancy, practice letting the pelvic floor muscles relax further, even bulge out slightly. This will give you the feeling of what you will have to do during labor to help the baby come out. Before you end the exercise, always tighten the muscles slightly.

Practice until the muscles begin to feel a little tired, and work up to doing five of these exercises at a time. Repeat about 10 times a day. You can practice them anywhere—on the bus, in the grocery line, at work, etc. Eventually, they will become a daily habit.

2 **Your Changing Feelings**

In this chapter, you will learn—

- ◆ How your emotions change during pregnancy.
- ◆ How sexuality is affected by pregnancy and how to stay close to your partner.
- ◆ About common worries during pregnancy and how to cope with them.
- ◆ How pregnancy and having a new baby in the family can change the expectations you and your partner have of each other and of your roles in the family.

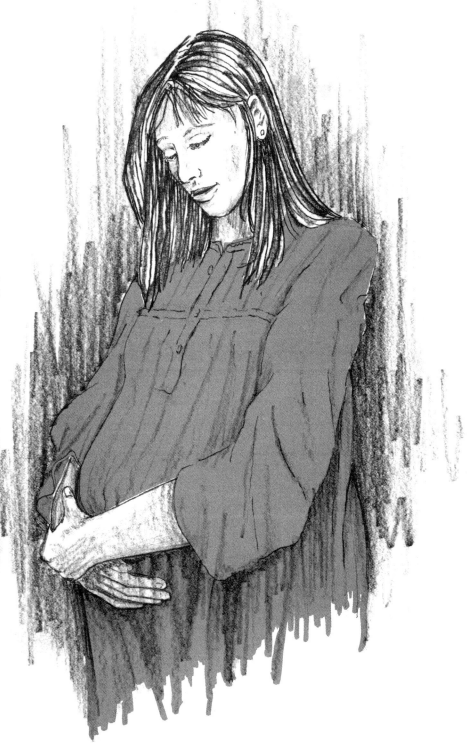

Your Changing Feelings

Expectant mothers and fathers may find that the emotional work of becoming a parent is nearly as great as the enormous physical changes the woman experiences. Being pregnant and dreaming of the baby that is coming is exciting. At the same time you may feel unsure of yourself or nervous about what lies ahead. Being pregnant affects not only your life and your partner's, but also your relationships with close friends and relatives. Your expectations of yourself and those around you may change and often this change is unsettling.

This chapter addresses the types of feelings you and your partner may experience during pregnancy, as well as questions you may have about sexuality, stress, and the changing expectations you and your partner may have of each other.

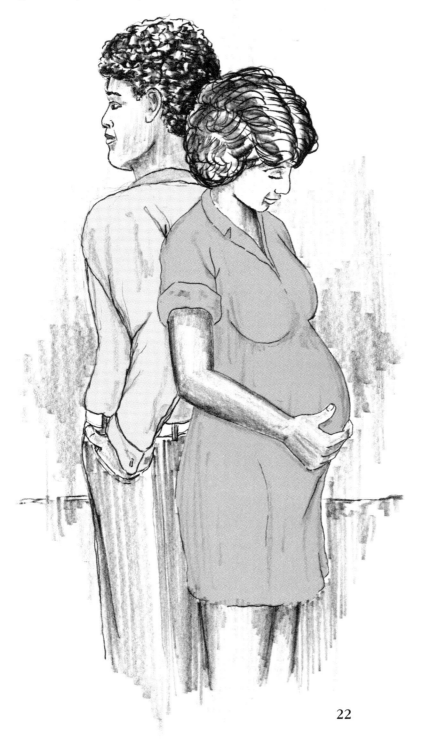

How Am I Feeling?

Use this think sheet to record your feelings and what you think you need from those around you. Have the baby's father do it too. You will have a chance to discuss what you have written during class. You will probably find that you and your classmates share many of the same feelings.

Mother's Feelings

_____

_____

_____

_____

_____

_____

What I Need

_____

_____

_____

_____

_____

_____

Father's Feelings

_____

_____

_____

_____

_____

_____

What I Need

_____

_____

_____

_____

_____

_____

Common Feelings and Needs of Expectant Mothers

Below is a list of feelings and needs that expectant mothers often have during pregnancy. It is normal to be both "up" and "down" about being pregnant, and the way you feel may change from day to day. After all, if this is your first pregnancy, you are finding your way through unfamiliar territory without a map.

Feelings	Needs
I can't believe I'm pregnant!	Time and space to rest.
Am I really ready to be a mother?	Reassurance from your partner that he loves and supports you.
I want to do the right things to take care of myself and the baby.	Support and companionship from other pregnant women or new mothers.
My partner wants to make love, but I'm scared we'll hurt the baby if we do.	Information and support from your health care provider.
I'm feeling much sexier now. Will my partner think I am now that my body has changed so much?	Accurate information on the stages of fetal development and childbirth.
I need someone to take care of me.	Reassurance that body changes are normal and the baby is okay.
I am so tired of being trapped in this big, awkward body.	Active childbirth preparation.
What will this baby be like?	
I dream and fantasize about the baby all the time now.	
I'm afraid my baby won't be normal.	
I can't wait to have the baby, but I'm afraid of going through labor.	
I'm going to miss feeling the baby inside me after he or she is born.	

Common Feelings and Needs of Expectant Fathers

As an expectant father, you may share some of the same feelings as your partner, but many of your feelings are different. You aren't experiencing all the hormonal and physical changes that she is, but your emotional adjustment to parenthood is just as complicated and wonderful. The feelings and needs below are common among expectant fathers and may help you understand and appreciate your own.

Feelings	Needs
I can't believe she's pregnant!	Her reassurance that you are loved, needed, and appreciated.
Am I really ready to be a father?	Support from family and friends, especially from other expectant fathers.
I want her to take good care of herself and the baby.	Information and support from her health care provider.
I'm scared I'll hurt the baby when we make love.	Accurate information on fetal development and prenatal care.
She's the one who's pregnant, but I'm gaining weight too.	Reassurance that her body changes are normal and that the baby is okay.
I envy all the attention she's getting now.	Active childbirth preparation.
I think her pregnant body is really beautiful.	
I worry that the baby won't be normal.	
I'm so worried about whether she'll be okay during delivery.	
What will happen if I can't help her during labor?	
I feel very strongly that I do (or do not) want to be in the delivery room when the baby is born.	

Is There Sex After Pregnancy?

Although sex obviously had everything to do with your being pregnant now, you and your partner may be surprised at how being pregnant changes your sexual relationship. People's levels of sexual desire change throughout a pregnancy, and every person responds to sexuality during pregnancy in a very personal way. Following are answers to some common questions that pregnant women and their partners ask about sex during pregnancy.

My partner and I worry about hurting the baby while we are having sex. Is this possible?

In most cases, intercourse is safe throughout a pregnancy. The baby is cushioned in the woman's body by the amniotic sac and protected from infection through the vagina by the mucous plug in the cervix. In certain pregnancies there may be medical reasons for restricting sexual activity due to risk of miscarriage or other health problems. If you are told to limit sexual activity, be sure to ask your health care provider what type of sexual activity—intercourse and/or orgasm—should be avoided.

How long will we be able to have sex?

In most cases, there is no medical reason not to have sex throughout your pregnancy. A personal decision about when to stop having intercourse should be tailored to each woman and man. Talk to your health care provider about what conditions apply to sex in your pregnancy.

Is it normal for a pregnant woman and her partner to feel really interested in sex sometimes and totally disinterested at other times?

Sexual interest during pregnancy goes through many ups and downs. In early pregnancy, the woman may feel less sexy due to morning sickness, tender breasts, mood swings, fatigue, irritability, and possibly anxiety over potential miscarriage. Even though there are real reasons for her being unavailable at this time, her partner may feel abandoned and left out.

In the second trimester, women may feel more like having sex. Initial discomforts have passed and certain physical and hormonal changes make her feel sexier. The man at this point may be able to respond to her renewed interest or he may be turned off by her increasing size and the obvious movement of the baby.

Many women become less interested in sexual intercourse during the last three months of pregnancy. A woman's increased size and her tendency to turn inward emotionally in preparation for the baby's arrival may lessen her sexual desire. Her partner may feel more or less turned on by her changed body and may also have his own share of anxiety about the birth of the baby and the changes that will occur in his life.

Throughout these changes, it is most important that you and your partner talk to each other about your feelings. If intercourse is not something one or both of you is interested in, try alternative ways of sexual expression or show affection for each other by a gentle massage. Staying close physically will help you cope with the stresses of pregnancy.

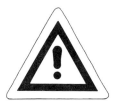

Note: Blowing air into the vagina of a pregnant woman can cause an air embolism (air bubble in the blood) that can result in death to the woman.

Worries and How to Cope

For many women, being pregnant is a stressful experience. The mixed feelings, mood swings, physical changes, and changes in your personal relationships can be unsettling. Being stressed during your pregnancy affects not only you but your baby. When you are stressed, the blood flow to the uterus is reduced so the baby receives less oxygen and has an increased heartbeat. A baby can handle this occasionally, but stress on a regular basis it is not good for you or your baby. Mothers with high levels of stress may have more problems during pregnancy and childbirth.

Although you will not be able to get rid of all the things that cause you to worry or be upset, there are many things you can do to deal with stress in a positive way. For example, talking to someone is often the first and best step. It could be your partner, a friend, a relative, a member of the clergy, or a professional counselor. Regular physical exercise and hobbies can help. Relaxation, meditation, and visualization are also well-known methods of stress management. (See Chapters 4 and 6.) Being in touch with your personal or spiritual beliefs will also help.

In all times of stress, it is important to eat well. A balanced diet helps keep your body strong and healthy and helps prevent illness. A combination of all these approaches might not rid you of all your stress, but it can improve your outlook.

Decisions

From the time you get pregnant, and maybe even before, you start to realize how many decisions have to be made when a baby joins your life. "What type of childbirth experience do I want?" "What will I name my baby?" "Where will the baby sleep?" "Will I work after the baby is born?" "Will I breastfeed or bottle feed my baby?" "Who will be my baby's health care provider?" These issues and many others will be decided by you during your pregnancy and after the baby arrives. One way of approaching the many decisions that you face and the stress that may go with them is to think about them and make some plans before the baby arrives.

You have just begun to think about your baby's birth and your expectations about labor and birth. In addition to your own wishes, the hospital and your health care provider may have their own policies and procedures for labor and birth. It is wise to begin considering the options available to you so that you feel confident about making a decision that is right for you. When you decide what you want, discuss it with your health care provider. If the options you want are not offered, try to reach a compromise.

Review the information in "Choices in Childbirth" in Appendix A. Other decisions you will need to make include those about infant feeding (see Chapter 8), circumcision (see Chapter 8), and returning to work (see Chapter 11 and "Child Care Choices" in Appendix B).

What Are You Worried About?

This think sheet lists common concerns that cause stress for expectant parents. Add any others that apply to your own situation. Then discuss them with your partner or with your class and see if you can come up with actions you can take to reduce the stress. Don't be afraid to ask others for help in managing stress.

Concerns	Actions I Can Take
Financial:	_____
____ not enough income	_____
____ baby clothing and equipment costs	_____
____ child care costs	_____
____ other _____	_____
Psychological:	_____
____ mood swings	_____
____ changes in relationships	_____
____ lack of support from family or friends	_____
____ other _____	_____
Physical (mother):	_____
____ body changes	_____
____ sexual behavior changes	_____
____ feeling trapped in a strange body	_____
____ feeling tired	_____
____ feeling nauseous	_____
____ not enough rest	_____
____ other _____	_____

Concerns	Actions I Can Take

Concerns

Actions I Can Take

Worries about the baby:

____ health

____ sex

____ abnormalities

____ other _____

Environmental:

____ excessive noise

____ limited space

____ cigarette smoke from others

____ other _____

Health care:

____ dislike health care provider

____ limited choices for prenatal care and
     delivery

____ costs

____ limited or no health insurance

____ other _____

Where to Go for Help

You may be eligible for financial assistance from local or federal government agencies. The federal government funds the Special Supplemental Food Program for Women, Infants, and Children, also known as WIC. WIC distributes specific nutritional foods and nutrition education to program participants—low-income, pregnant women; postpartum and breastfeeding women; and children up to age five who are in need of nutritional help.

Another federal program, the Expanded Food and Nutrition Education Program (EFNEP), provides advice and assistance to people who qualify based on income. You can get more information on EFNEP from state and local offices of the Extension Service in your area.

Local public health clinics can give you more information on applying for assistance under WIC and EFNEP. Other assistance may be available from local social service agencies and churches. Your childbirth class instructor, clergy member, or health care provider may be able to help you locate the nearest offices of these agencies.

If you are a member of the U.S. military living overseas, these services and programs are not available to you. See "Resources for Overseas Military Personnel and Their Dependents" in Appendix C for a list of social services available overseas.

For Single Mothers

If you will be a single mother, you and all others interested in you may have special concerns about your pregnancy. You may find yourself feeling alone in your pregnancy or you may be getting too much unwanted advice from friends and relatives. Financial pressures are likely to be more intense for you now and after the baby is born. Your instructor may be able to suggest social service agencies in your community that can help you.

All pregnant women must manage stress to ensure their health and that of their baby. This is even more true for an expectant mother who is single, divorced, or widowed. Taking responsibility for the health and safety of yourself and your baby is one of the most important things you will do in life. It can also be one of your most enriching and satisfying experiences.

For Teen Mothers

Being a teenager and being pregnant puts a double strain on your body and emotions. During your teen years you undergo enormous physical and emotional changes. These changes are almost as great as those changes that occur during pregnancy. The changes of pregnancy combined with the changes of the teenage years put demands on your body and emotions that older pregnant women do not experience.

You are probably living at home with your family, and you may or may not have their support. Your friends may be more interested in their busy, active lives than in your pregnancy. Your relationship with the baby's father may have changed too since the pregnancy, and you may feel very isolated and alone.

Even though your need for support is great and the changes very scary, don't let fear control you. Something wonderful is happening inside of you, and you can make many choices that will produce the best possible outcome for you and your baby. It is important for you to focus on your own health and that of your baby. You can do this by eating right, thinking positively, exercising, relaxing, and getting good health care. Make a special effort during this time to make changes for the better. This will help you view your pregnancy positively.

Being responsible for a healthy pregnancy will give you confidence and understanding about the ways your choices affect your life. Whether you decide to keep the baby or to release the baby for adoption, treat yourself very specially and with care. You deserve only the best right now! Taking care of yourself during pregnancy is the best gift you will ever give to your baby and yourself.

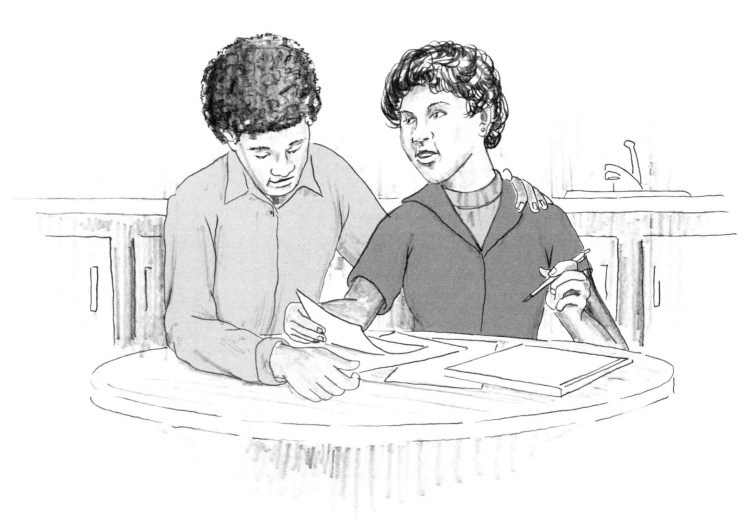

Changing Family Roles

The process of becoming a parent begins at the moment of conception. During the nine months of pregnancy, expectant mothers and fathers begin to view themselves, each other, and family members in new ways. It is important for expectant mothers and fathers to be clear with each other about how they expect to share household and baby-care responsibilities after the baby is born. In most cases, changes will have to be made when the baby arrives and there will be some stress involved until new roles become comfortable and familiar.

Having a child will create new responsibilities for everyone involved and will complicate decision making on a personal and family level. Because your time and financial resources will be affected by having a baby, you will be called on to make careful choices about setting priorities.

The following think sheets give you a chance to explore your expectations about family roles. There are no right or wrong answers to any of the questions. They are designed to help you clarify your thoughts and communicate with your partner. You and your partner should fill out the think sheet without talking to each other. When you have both finished, compare your answers and discuss them.

Family Roles: Mother

Below is a list of common household and infant-care tasks. Give each one a number from 1 to 10 based on whether you feel the task is something a mother always does, a father always does, something a mother and father equally share responsibility for, or something in between. If a task does not apply to your situation, don't give it a number. Without consulting your partner, rate each task. Then have your partner do the same on the other side of this page. After you have both finished, compare your answers.

Mother Always Does				Both Mother and Father Do				Father Always Does	
1	2	3	4	5	6	7	8	9	10

____ Keep the house clean.

____ Take out the trash.

____ Do the grocery shopping.

____ Do other shopping (clothes, household appliances, etc.)

____ Plan and cook the meals.

____ Diaper the baby.

____ Bathe the baby.

____ Feed the baby.

____ Feed and take care of pets.

____ Wash the dishes.

____ Take care of household repairs.

____ Take the baby to the clinic for well-baby and sick visits.

____ Wash the clothes.

____ Balance the checkbook. Manage the family budget.

____ Maintain the family automobile.

____ Work to support the family.

____ Find a babysitter so you and your partner can have time alone.

Family Roles: Father

Below is a list of common household and infant-care tasks. Give each one a number from 1 to 10 based on whether you feel the task is something a mother always does, a father always does, something a mother and father equally share responsibility for, or something in between. If a task does not apply to your situation, don't give it a number. Without consulting your partner, rate each task. Your partner should have already done the same on the other side of this page. After you have both finished, compare your answers.

Mother Always Does				Both Mother and Father Do				Father Always Does
1	2	3	4	5	6	7	8	9	10

____ Keep the house clean.

____ Take out the trash.

____ Do the grocery shopping.

____ Do other shopping (clothes, household appliances, etc.)

____ Plan and cook the meals.

____ Diaper the baby.

____ Bathe the baby.

____ Feed the baby.

____ Feed and take care of pets.

____ Wash the dishes.

____ Take care of household repairs.

____ Take the baby to the clinic for well-baby and sick visits.

____ Wash the clothes.

____ Balance the checkbook. Manage the family budget.

____ Maintain the family automobile.

____ Work to support the family.

____ Find a babysitter so you and your partner can have time alone.

3 How Your Baby Grows

In this chapter, you will learn—
- How your baby develops inside the womb.
- What to eat during pregnancy.
- What substances to avoid or limit during pregnancy.
- How to prevent injuries.

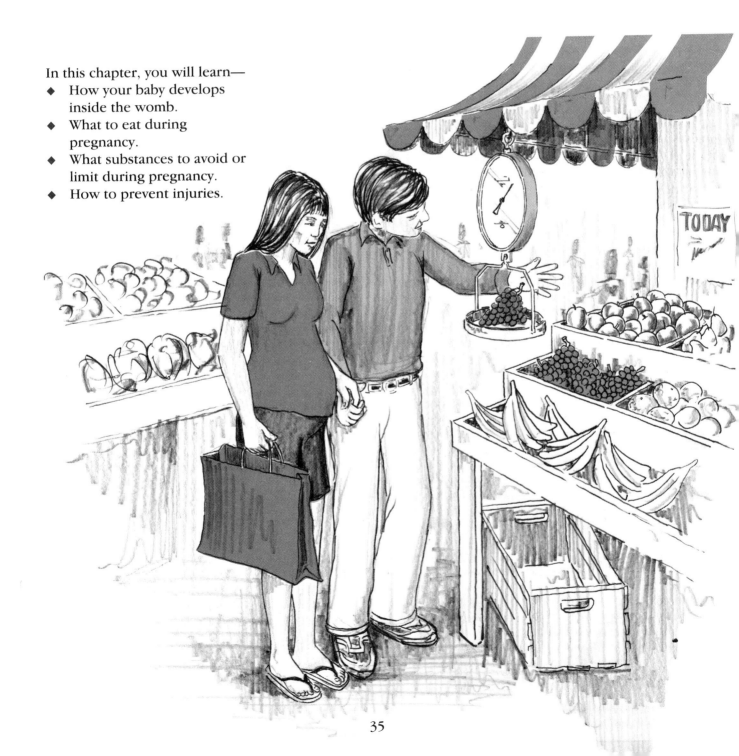

The growth of your baby is a miracle happening. From the tiny embryo to the nine-month-old fetus, your baby lives and develops, protected inside of you. What you eat, drink, and think about, along with the situations and substances you avoid during pregnancy, will make a difference in the health and well-being of your child.

Your Baby Month by Month

You may wonder how your baby grows inside of you. Here is a month-by-month account:

◆ **Conception**—About 14 days after a menstrual period, a single egg leaves one of your ovaries and begins to move down the fallopian tube. If it is fertilized by a sperm after sexual intercourse, the egg goes through a series of changes over the next few days. The cell begins to divide. Soon a ball of cells forms and moves farther down the fallopian tube to the uterus. There it begins to embed itself into the uterus, getting food and oxygen from your bloodstream.

Note: Even though conception takes place about 14 days after a menstrual period, it is usual to date a pregnancy from the first day of your last period, not from when you actually conceived the baby. Therefore your baby is usually two weeks old at the end of the first month of pregnancy.

First Trimester

◆ **First month**—The baby's brain begins to form in the first month. At the end of the third week, the baby's first body organs form. Blood starts to circulate by the third week. At the end of the third week, the baby is about one-eighth of an inch long with a heart and developing nervous, skeletal, and digestive systems. At this stage the baby is called an embryo.

◆ **Second month**—The baby is now about two inches long and weighs one-third of an ounce. During this time, all major organ systems develop. The eyes begin to form. The arms and legs take shape. The nose begins to

form. The brain grows quickly. The placenta, which takes nutrients from your body for the baby, begins to form.

◆ **Third month**—Calcium begins to be deposited in the baby's bones and continues to be deposited throughout pregnancy. The baby begins to move: kicking legs, waving arms, swallowing amniotic fluid. The baby has lips and a tongue. By 12 weeks the baby is about three inches long and weighs one-half of an ounce. The formation of all major body parts is complete by the 13th week.

Second Trimester

◆ **Fourth month**—The baby's skin looks pink and transparent. The baby will increase his or her weight by six times during this month. The eyelids are still shut, but the eyes are forming.

◆ **Fifth month**—The baby is almost 12 inches long and weighs about one-half pound. You could tell now by looking whether the baby is a girl or a boy. This is when you will begin to feel your baby move (this is called quickening), first as a flutter and then as thumps and bumps. Eyelashes and eyebrows appear.

◆ **Sixth month**—The baby is now covered with a creamy substance called vernix, which protects the baby's skin inside the uterus. You may notice that the baby responds to loud noises and music. The baby is usually very active when you are resting! The baby stretches, kicks, and sucks his or her thumb. Hair is forming on top of the baby's head.

Third Trimester

◆ **Seventh month**—The baby is 14 to 17 inches long and weighs 2-1/2 to 3 pounds. She or he is gaining fat. Babies born at 28 weeks have a 60 to 70 percent chance of survival, but they require intensive care to survive. They are better off inside the womb until they are at least 38 weeks. The baby continues to suck his or her thumb and swallows amniotic fluid in preparation for eating after birth.

- **Eighth month**—The baby continues to grow rapidly and gain fat. The lungs continue to mature. You may feel the baby hiccuping (it feels like regular, jerky movements inside). The last trimester is the time of greatest brain and nervous system growth. During this month the baby will gain about two pounds.
- **Ninth month**—The baby is ready to be born. She or he is 20 to 22 inches long and weighs about seven pounds. She or he may not move as much because there is less room to do so. The baby can see, hear, move, cry, suck, and swallow.

Eating Well for You and Your Baby

Eating well during pregnancy is one of the most important gifts you can give to your baby. All nutrients and fluids come to your baby through your bloodstream by way of the placenta. Needs for almost every nutrient increase during pregnancy to take care of the growth and development of the baby and to meet your increased needs.

The chart beginning on page 38 contains the recommended servings of the foods that you should be eating each day during pregnancy. Take a few minutes to write down everything you ate yesterday. Using the food groups listed in the chart, count how many servings you had of each group and fill in the blanks in the column on the right. How did you do?

What I ate yesterday

_____

_____

_____

_____

_____

How many servings I had yesterday

_____ Dairy

_____ Protein

_____ Fruits and vegetables

_____ Breads and cereals

What to Eat When You Are Pregnant

Needs	How Much	What It Gives You and the Baby
Dairy Group		
Milk group: whole, skim, powdered, canned, buttermilk also: cottage cheese, white cheese, yellow cheese, yogurt, ice cream, and other foods made with milk	4 servings (1 serving is: 1–1/2 cups cottage cheese or 1–1/2 slices of cheese or 1 cup of milk or 1 cup of yogurt.)	Calcium: needed for strong bones and teeth; helps nerves and muscles work well Protein: the building block of the body; important for recovery after delivery Vitamin D: helps the body use calcium Vitamin A: needed for eyes, skin, hair, and body growth
Protein Group		
Meat and other protein foods: meat, fish, chicken, eggs, liver also: pinto beans, dried peas, nuts, soybeans, peanut butter, tofu	3 servings (1 serving is: 2–3 oz. of meat [the size of the back of your hand] or 2 eggs or 3/4 cup of cooked beans or 1/4 cup of peanut butter or 1/2 cup of nuts.)	Protein: building block of the body; needed to build strong tissues and keep them healthy; important for recovery after birth Folic acid: B vitamin needed to help body use iron Iron: needed for red blood cells, which carry oxygen through the body; prevents anemia B vitamins: needed for healthy nerves; helps body use other nutrients

What to Eat When You Are Pregnant

Needs	How Much	What It Gives You and the Baby
Fruits and Vegetables Group		
Fruits: Oranges, grapefruits, melons, strawberries, tangerines, apples, apricots, plums, peaches, bananas, grapes, nectarines, etc.	4 servings of fruits and vegetables Include 1 citrus or other vitamin C fruit (1 serving is: an average size piece of fruit or a melon wedge or 6 oz. of fruit juice or 1/2 cup of berries or 1/4 cup of sliced or cooked fruit or 1/4 cup of dried fruit.)	Vitamin C: helps keep body healthy; needed for teeth, gums, bones, body cells, and blood vessels Vitamin A: needed for eyes, skin, hair, normal growth
Vegetables: Dark green or deep yellow vegetables Dark green: beet greens, broccoli, collard greens, kale, mustard greens, spinach, turnip greens, etc. Deep yellow: carrots, pumpkin, sweet potato, winter squash Other: beets, cabbage, cauliflower, celery, Chinese cabbage, cucumber, green beans, etc.	(1 serving is: 1/2 cup of cooked or cut-up vegetables or 1 cup of raw leafy vegetables.)	Vitamin A Vitamin C Fiber: needed for proper digestion

What to Eat When You Are Pregnant

Needs	How Much	What It Gives You and the Baby
Bread and Cereal Group		
Grains, breads, and cereals: whole-grain or enriched breads, cereal, muffins, tortillas, rice, pasta	4 or more servings (1 serving is: a slice of bread or 1/2 cup of cooked cereal, rice, or pasta or 1 oz. of ready-to-eat cereal or a small roll, muffin, or biscuit.)	Protein, starch, vitamins and minerals, fiber
Fats and Sweets Group		
Butter, margarine, mayonnaise, salad dressings, oils, candy, cakes, honey, jam, jelly, sherbet, soft drinks, gelatin deserts, or jellied salads		No nutrients, just flavor and calories

Questions About Nutrition in Pregnancy

Should I stop eating salt?
Some salt is necessary in every diet to help regulate fluid levels in the body. Usually it is not necessary to limit salt severely, but cutting down on foods like potato chips, processed meats (salami, bologna, etc.), and other foods high in sodium (salt) is a good health habit in general.

I can't drink milk. How can I get the calcium I need?
Some women are "lactose intolerant," which means they cannot drink milk or eat other dairy products. Other women just don't like the taste of milk. Additional sources of calcium are cheese, yogurt, cottage cheese, tofu, and some green vegetables. Unfortunately, it often takes a larger serving of these foods to get the calcium you need. If you really don't think you can get the calcium you need from your diet, talk to your health care provider about taking calcium supplements.

I eat in fast-food restaurants a lot. Can I get the foods I need when I eat there?
Just as at home or at the grocery store, there are good and bad choices that you can make. Salads are a good choice, as are juices and milk (as opposed to sodas). Baked potatoes are good, and so is chili. The chart on page 42 can help you make the best choices.

Is it true that if I eat strawberries, my baby will have a birthmark on his or her face?
No. All cultures have tales about foods that are considered dangerous to eat during pregnancy. Foods that are good for you are good for your baby.

My health care provider gave me iron tablets and vitamins to take. The iron makes me constipated. Also, I wonder if I should take more vitamins because I don't eat very well.
Iron tablets sometimes make constipation worse, but they are important because it is very hard to get enough iron from your diet during pregnancy. Drinking lots of water, eating fresh fruits and vegetables, and exercising regularly will help to relieve constipation.

Never take more vitamins or different vitamins than your health care provider prescribes without checking with your health care provider. Some vitamins can be dangerous to your baby if taken in excess amounts.

I'm a vegetarian. Is that a problem during pregnancy?
In general, if you are a vegetarian who eats dairy products and eggs, you should have no trouble getting the nutrition you need during pregnancy. If you eat no animal products at all, you may want to see a nutritional counselor to make sure you get the iron, folic acid, and protein you need. Protein can be obtained from many sources, such as tofu, beans, rice, and vegetables. You may have to take iron and folic acid supplements, but check with your health care provider first.

Making Fast Food Good Food

If you choose to eat in a fast-food restaurant, consider the following chart to help you make better choices. Fast-food restaurants are not recommended for daily eating. Homemade foods are cheaper and usually healthier.

Choose These	Instead of These
Baked potato, coleslaw, salad (limit dressings)	French fries, onion rings, potato puffs
Roast beef sandwich, lean ground beef	Hamburger with special sauces
Roasted chicken, grilled chicken, taco, chili, pizza	Fried chicken
Taco salad without sour cream, cheese, and chips	Nachos
Broiled seafood	Fried fish sandwich, breaded clams
Frozen yogurt	Sundaes, cookies, ice cream, pies, etc.
Fruit juices, low-fat milk	Soda, chocolate milk, coffee
Soups	

You are having dinner at your favorite fast-food restaurant. You ate a nutritious breakfast, not much for lunch, and you are starving. What could you order that would taste good and provide the best nutrition for you and your baby?

_____

_____

_____

_____

Be Good to Your Baby

Almost everything you take into your body passes from your placenta to the baby through the umbilical cord. Just because your body can tolerate certain amounts of some substances doesn't mean your baby's can. There are many substances that can harm your baby during pregnancy, and they should be avoided in any amount.

Listed below are the most common substances you should avoid, what effects they have, and alternative choices if you are having a hard time giving them up.

Substance
Cigarettes

How much is okay?
None

Effects on your baby
When an expectant mother smokes, the baby gets less nutrients and oxygen for growth and development, as well as many chemicals that affect him or her in many ways. Mothers who smoke have a higher risk of giving birth to smaller babies (who don't do as well as normal-weight babies) and premature babies, of having miscarriages and stillbirths, and of having babies who have respiratory problems at birth. Mothers who do not smoke but are exposed often to the cigarette smoke of others incur some of these risks as well.

What you can do
Stop smoking. Pick a quit day. When you feel like smoking, relax, take some deep breaths and try to think about why you want to quit. Think about your baby inside. Exercise every day if it's okay with your health care provider. Keep busy. Join a "quit smoking" group. Stay out of smoke-filled rooms as much as possible. Ask other smokers not to smoke around you. Try counseling or hypnosis. Avoid socializing with people who smoke.

For Fathers
If you smoke, stop now. This is a gift you can give to your baby. Babies and children who have parents who smoke have more colds, flu, bronchitis, and asthma. If you don't know how to stop, seek professional help. In the meantime, try to smoke outside or in a room away from your pregnant partner.

Substance
Alcohol

How much is okay?
None

Effects on your baby
Expectant mothers who are heavy drinkers sometimes have babies who suffer from fetal alcohol syndrome (FAS). These babies may have slow growth, mental retardation, heart problems, learning problems, and problems with other body systems. Even women who drink small-to-moderate amounts during pregnancy risk effects such as having a baby of small size, poor growth after birth, and lower intelligence. Moderate drinking is also associated with miscarriages and stillbirths.

What you can do
Stop drinking. Talk with your health care provider. If you use alcohol to relax or to stop being depressed, think of other ways to cope. Can you talk to someone who will listen to you? Sometimes exercise, relaxing music, or finding a way to vent your frustrations will help. If you feel you cannot stop drinking, go to Alcoholics Anonymous (AA) or another community self-help group.

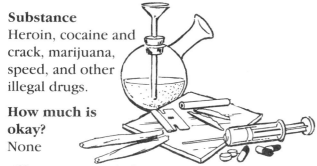

Substance
Heroin, cocaine and crack, marijuana, speed, and other illegal drugs.

How much is okay?
None

Effects on your baby
Babies born to mothers who use **heroin** may be smaller than normal or premature. They go through withdrawal after birth, which is painful and dangerous for them. They also may develop more slowly than other babies.

Cocaine and crack cut down on the supply of oxygen to the baby, which can retard the baby's growth and even cause the baby to have a stroke in the womb. They can also cause serious birth defects and brain damage. Babies born to mothers who use cocaine and crack often have trouble feeding, are irritable, and have tremors. They also have a higher rate of sudden infant death syndrome (SIDS). Long-term effects may include learning problems and behavior problems that last throughout life.

Marijuana, like cigarettes, robs the baby of nutrients and oxygen. Use of marijuana during pregnancy has been associated with miscarriages and other problems before birth, as well as with learning problems after birth.

What you can do
Stop using illegal drugs. Get help if you need it. Talk with your health care provider. Drugs can kill your baby!

Substance
Prescription medications

How much is okay?
Only as directed by your health care provider who knows you are pregnant.

Effects on your baby
Different medications have different effects on the baby, such as birth defects, discoloration of teeth, mental retardation.

What you can do
Don't take any medication unless you absolutely need to for your own health or the health of the baby. Always inform any health care provider that you are pregnant.

Some medications—such as drugs for diabetes (insulin), for thyroid problems, and to prevent seizures—are necessary, and the risks of not taking them may be greater than the risk of taking them.

Substance
Over-the-counter medications

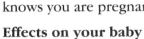

How much is okay?
Only as directed by your health care provider who knows you are pregnant.

Effects on your baby
Over-the-counter medications have various effects, depending on the medication. For example, aspirin should not be taken during pregnancy because it can cause bleeding problems for you or your baby. Some cold relief medications may be harmful to your baby. Even vitamins taken in the wrong amounts can be harmful, so take only what your health care provider prescribes.

What you can do
Take medication only after checking with your health care provider. Take medication only if absolutely needed. Try other solutions to aches and pains: for a headache, lie down and put a cool washcloth on your forehead; for a cold, drink lots of liquids, rest, and use a cool-water vaporizer.

Substance
Caffeine (found in tea, soft drinks, and chocolate, as well as in coffee)

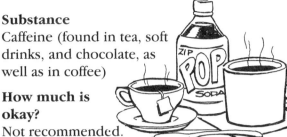

How much is okay?
Not recommended.

Effects on your baby
Caffeine causes the baby to have an increased heart rate and breathing rate. The effects are uncertain, but caution is indicated.

What you can do
Switch to decaffeinated coffee, tea, and soft drinks. Drink more water and juices.

Healthy Habits

Choose one or two health changes that you would like to make during pregnancy. Think about what keeps you from making these changes. Then think about what would help you to make the changes and include the names of people who can help you.

At the end, make a brief statement of your goal, such as "I will eat a green salad and drink four glasses of milk every day" or "I will exercise three times a week."

Health changes I would like to make

_____

_____

What keeps me from changing?

_____

_____

Ideas for making changes

_____

_____

My goal

_____

_____

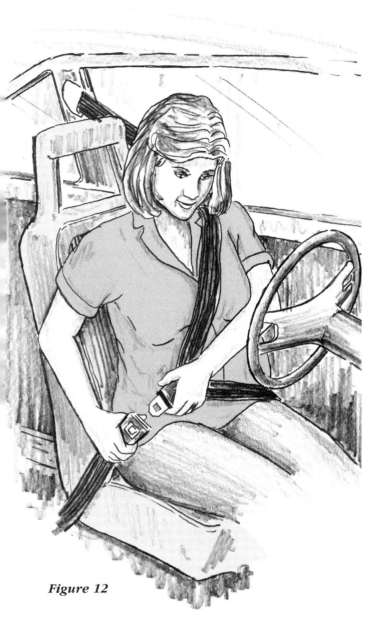

Figure 12

A Safe Pregnancy

The fact that you are pregnant means that you must pay attention to the way your everyday life affects you and your baby. Your changing shape sometimes makes activities that you have always taken for granted more difficult and tiring, and potentially risky. Your baby may be exposed to chemicals, radiation, or infections at work and at home that may be harmful. Listed below are some general tips on preventing injuries, as well as some specific suggestions about what to avoid at home and in the workplace.

Preventing Injuries

Contrary to what many people think, most injuries are preventable. Here are some simple steps that you can take to prevent injuries to yourself and your baby:

♦ As your center of gravity shifts because of the weight of the baby, it's more difficult to keep your balance. Take things more slowly and be careful when climbing steps and ladders.

♦ Wear low heels or flats to decrease back strain and to avoid being thrown off balance.

♦ Be careful getting in and out of the tub.

♦ Wear auto safety belts at all times. Make sure the lap belt is positioned under your abdomen at the level of the pubic bone, and always use a shoulder strap. If you have automatic belts, make sure you wear the lap belt also *(Fig. 12)*.

♦ Don't travel with any driver who has been drinking.

♦ Avoid back injury at home and on the job by using good posture and by lifting only from a knees-bent position.

♦ During the first trimester, nausea, dizziness, fatigue, and heat sensitivity increase the risks of injuries. Be careful!

♦ At the end of pregnancy, the body's changes may cause increased risks of falls, and normal physical activity may be more tiring. Be careful!

♦ Check your workplace and home for substances that may be harmful to your baby.

Disease and Infection

Some diseases and infections you can catch from other people are hazardous to your baby during pregnancy. You should do your best to avoid exposure to disease and infection including those discussed below:

◆ **Sexually transmitted diseases (STDs)** can be hazardous to a pregnant woman and/or her baby. Common STDs are gonorrhea, syphilis, chlamydia, genital herpes, and HIV (the virus that causes AIDS). **If you think you have been exposed to or have an STD, contact your health care provider immediately.** If you have been exposed to an STD, you also may be interested in seeking counseling on how best to deal with the situation.

Gonorrhea, syphilis, and chlamydia can be treated with antibiotics. Injury to the baby may be prevented if they are diagnosed early. A baby infected with genital herpes at birth can be severely brain-damaged. For that reason, women who have active herpes lesions during labor should have a cesarean delivery. This reduces the risk of infection to the baby, but it does not prevent it.

When a woman is infected with HIV, it can infect the baby even if she has no symptoms of the disease. Many people are infected and don't know it. People can become infected with HIV by—

  ◆ Sharing needles and syringes with someone who has the virus.
  ◆ Having sex with someone who has the virus.
  ◆ Receiving a blood transfusion with the virus.

HIV cannot be caught from toilet seats or casual contact.

Using a condom during intercourse provides some protection against contracting and spreading STDs.

◆ **Infections** can be dangerous to a pregnant woman and/or her baby. If you have been around anyone with German measles (rubella), chicken pox, or other viruses, call your health care provider. German measles can cause a baby to be deaf or retarded. Try to avoid being around anyone with an infection.

◆ **Hepatitis B** is a viral infection that is dangerous to a pregnant woman and her baby. It is transmitted through blood or blood by-products, saliva, vaginal secretions, or semen. It can be transmitted to the baby. People at risk for hepatitis B are drug abusers who use needles and their sexual partners, sexual partners of people with hepatitis B, people who have received blood or blood by-products, and health care personnel. Anyone in these high-risk groups should be tested for this virus.

◆ **Toxoplasmosis** is a disease carried by cats and other animals. Toxoplasmosis is usually harmless, but it can cause birth defects. If you have a cat, have someone else change the litter and handle the cat. It's a good idea to wear gloves when digging in the soil outside, in case other cats have used your garden as a litter box. If you have a cat, your health care provider may wish to test you for toxoplasmosis. The disease can also be transmitted through raw or very rare meat, so avoid eating these.

Hazards

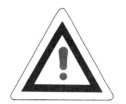

X rays: Tell any dentist or doctor you visit that you are pregnant. X rays are not recommended during pregnancy because they could harm the baby. If X rays of your upper body are necessary, your abdomen should be protected with a lead apron.

Hazards in the Workplace:

Heavy metals—lead and mercury

Radiation—X rays and exposure to radioisotopes

Anesthetic gases—such as those in an operating room and a dentist's office

Hazards at Home:

Chemical cleaners—such as oven cleaners

Pesticides and insecticides

Paint and paint removers

Note: Always read labels before using such products.

Lead—Lead hazards may be hidden in your home: in paint, in dust, in drinking water, and in the soil. Avoid removing old paint and don't let anyone else remove old paint while you are pregnant. To avoid ingesting lead dust, wash your hands before eating or preparing food. Use a wet mop or sponge to clean floors and woodwork. If possible, have your water tested.

4 *Enjoying Pregnancy*

In this chapter, you will learn—
◆ About the importance of physical exercise.
◆ How to relax and the benefits of relaxation.
◆ How to visualize and the benefits of visualization.

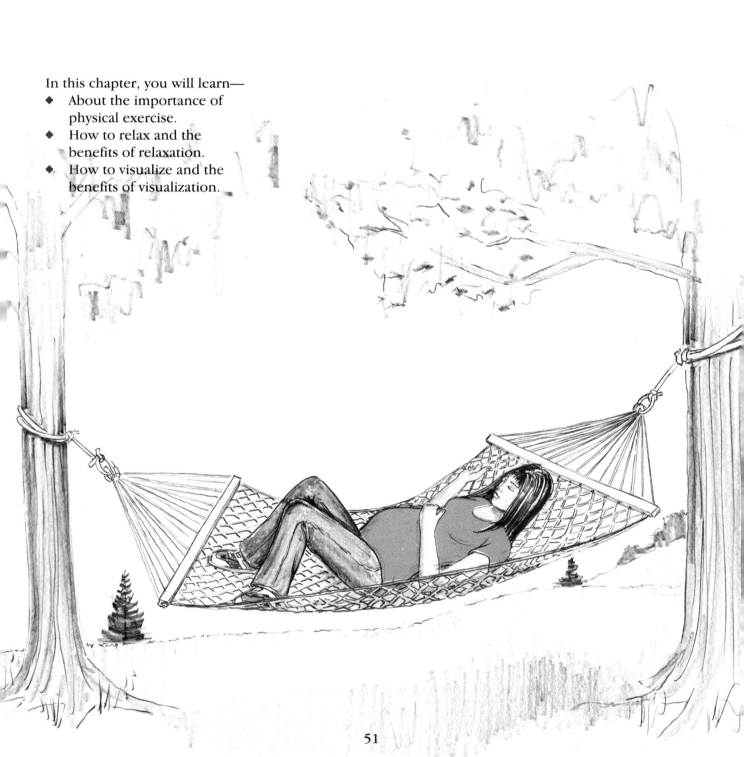

Pregnancy is a time to take care of yourself and to learn not to worry about the little things. In this chapter, you will learn skills for coping with stress: exercise, relaxation, and visualization. Exercise can make you more comfortable, help you get in shape, and keep up your energy. Relaxation skills can be used throughout pregnancy, labor and birth, and parenthood. In this session, you will practice progressive relaxation. It is a simple yet effective way to relax all of your muscles. Visualization is another tool you can use for taking care of yourself, and you will practice a simple visualization. These stress-reducing techniques promote positive thinking and well-being now and after your baby is born. Use them throughout your life to make yourself feel good.

Exercise and Fitness During Pregnancy

A lot of people don't exercise because they think it's too hard or too boring, or maybe because they have never tried. But here are some of the reasons why it's good to exercise during pregnancy:

◆ It feels good.
◆ It's fun.
◆ It makes you look good.
◆ It gives you more energy.
◆ It makes you more comfortable during pregnancy.
◆ It helps to get you in shape for labor.
◆ It helps you get back in shape faster after the pregnancy.

Basically, when you exercise, you feel better about yourself and more in control of your life.

Note: Always check with your health care provider before you begin any exercise program.

What Exercises to Do

Pregnancy is not the time to start a new intense exercise program. Begin with something you are doing already or know how to do. Swimming and brisk walking are probably the best exercises to do during pregnancy. Other activities, such as dancing, can also provide good exercise. Even if you had not exercised before you became pregnant, you can still start with something like a walking program that begins slowly and builds up to 15 minutes a day, three or four times a week. You also can ride a stationary bike.

If you were jogging regularly before you became pregnant, you can usually continue at a lesser pace (see the safety guidelines on the next page), but you should talk to your health care provider first.

Stretching is always important to do before you exercise or just as an exercise itself. It will keep you limber and help prevent injuries. When you stretch, always do it gently to get the maximum benefit. Bouncing or jerky movements can hurt you.

If you decide to exercise regularly, make an exercise schedule and stick to it. You'll feel a sense of accomplishment and receive health and fitness benefits.

Take a couple of minutes to write down your ideas about exercise below.

Types of exercise I like to do

_____

_____

Why I like to do them

_____

_____

When I can do them

_____

_____

How exercise makes me feel

_____

_____

52

Safety Guidelines for Exercise During Pregnancy

Following are some guidelines to follow to help you exercise safely during pregnancy:

- ◆ Regular exercise (three or more times a week) is better than occasional exercise.
- ◆ Don't exercise outdoors in hot, humid weather.
- ◆ Avoid jerky, bouncy motions.
- ◆ Stretch gently; avoid overstretching.
- ◆ Warm up for five minutes before and cool down after each exercise session.
- ◆ Each exercise session (not including times for warm-up and cool-down) should not be more than 15 minutes.
- ◆ Measure your heart rate, making sure you don't go over 140 beats per minute.

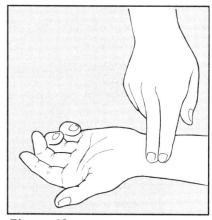

Figure 13

How to Measure Your Heart Rate

To measure your heart rate, turn your hand palm up. Place the index and middle fingers of your other hand near the thumb side of the wrist *(Fig. 13)*. Count the beats of the pulse for six seconds and multiply by 10. This is your heartbeat per minute.

- ◆ Drink water before and after you exercise.
- ◆ Always stop if you have any pain, dizziness, nausea, or shortness of breath. If any of these symptoms persist after you stop exercising, call your health care provider.
- ◆ If you experience vaginal bleeding or uterine contractions, call your health care provider immediately.

Relaxation

There are many ways to relax: deep breathing, meditation, progressive relaxation, music, massage. In this session, you will practice progressive relaxation. In Module II, you will practice other relaxation methods that are especially helpful in labor and birth. Begin to explore how you relax the best—that is often an indication of what will be most helpful to you in labor.

You should use relaxation skills when—

◆ You are tired.
◆ Your back aches and your shoulders are tight.
◆ You can't sleep at night.
◆ You are tempted to go back to bad habits, such as smoking, drinking, or eating junk food to reduce tension.
◆ The demands of job, house, or family get to you.

Relaxation skills will help you—

◆ Manage your stress.
◆ Feel more comfortable.
◆ Think more clearly.

One way to relax is just to do some slow, deep breathing. First, take a deep breath in through your nose and let out a big sigh through your mouth. As you breathe in the second time, think to yourself "relax." As you breathe out, feel that you are breathing out all the tension in your body. Do this several times. Take this relaxation break many times during the day.

Another way to relax is **progressive relaxation**—the deep relaxation of muscle groups. Practice the following progressive relaxation exercise in class and use it at home. Practice often. The more you practice, the easier it gets.

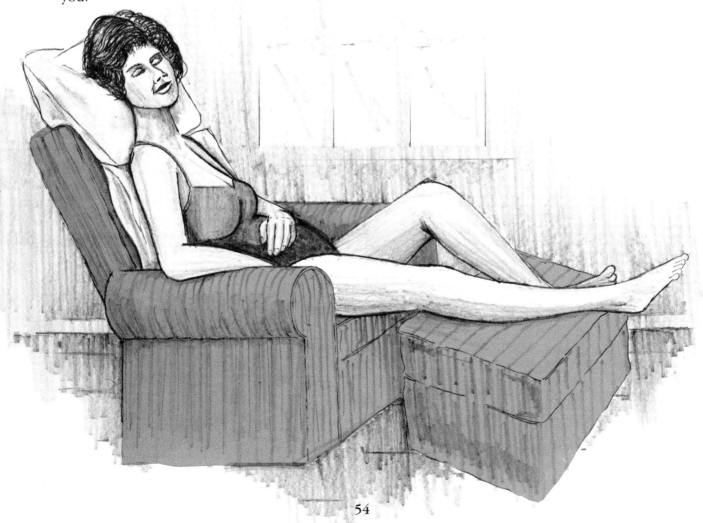

Progressive Relaxation Practice Sheet

Find a comfortable position, either lying on your side with many pillows or in a comfortable chair. If you are comfortable only on your back, be sure to prop several pillows or place a wedge under your head and shoulders. Close your eyes. Begin to breathe slowly and easily, in and out.

◆

Focus on your face. Tense your face by clenching your jaw, wrinkling your forehead, and squeezing your eyes tightly shut. Then relax completely, all at once. Feel your jaw become slack, your brow more smooth, and your eyelids more relaxed.

◆

Focus on your left arm and hand. Tense your left arm and hand by clenching your left fist tightly. Relax completely, all at once. Allow your arm to go limp. Feel a warm sensation in your fingertips as you become deeply relaxed.

◆

Tense your right arm and hand by clenching your right fist tightly. Relax completely, all at once. Allow your arm to go limp. Again, feel a warm sensation in your fingertips as you become deeply relaxed.

◆

Focus on your breathing. Imagine breathing in relaxation, and breathing out tension. Make it slow and comfortable, and remind yourself that this is your time to relax. Just let go.

◆

Focus on your neck and shoulders. Tense your neck and shoulders. Then relax completely, all at once. Allow your shoulders to drop comfortably and your neck to relax.

◆

Focus on your breathing, breathing in relaxation and breathing out tension.

◆

Focus on your chest, back, and stomach. Tense these areas by tightening your stomach, pressing your back into the floor or the chair, and tightening your buttocks. Then relax completely, all at once. Let yourself sink back comfortably into the floor or the chair.

◆

Focus on your breathing, breathing in relaxation and breathing out tension.

◆

Focus on your right leg and foot. Think about how they feel. Tense your right leg and foot by raising them slightly off the floor and pointing your toes toward your nose. Then relax completely, all at once. Let your thigh and calf muscles relax. Feel your toes get warm.

◆

Focus on your left leg and foot. Think about how they feel. Now, tense your left leg and foot by raising them slightly off the floor and pointing your toes toward your nose. Then relax completely, all at once. Let your thigh and calf muscles relax. Feel your toes get warm.

◆

Take a few minutes to make a mental check down your body. Think about where you still feel tension. As you breathe out, release this tension. Notice if you feel any difference.

◆

Slowly begin to wake up your body. Wiggle your fingers and toes. Move your arms and legs gently. Open your eyes. When you are ready, sit up very slowly.

Creative Visualization

What is creative visualization?

Creative visualization is a means of translating positive thoughts into mental images or pictures. It means seeing and feeling a desired result with your eyes closed. You can use visualization to create positive things in your life. Whenever you imagine something, you are using your creative abilities to "visualize" an idea in your mind. If you focus on this idea to create a clear image of what you want, then it's called creative visualization. It is using the power of your imagination to achieve a goal. Creative visualization exercises may be guided by someone else or self-guided.

Who uses it?

Anyone can use creative visualization. In fact, you use it every day when you think or imagine things. When you add a sense of purpose to it, then you are creatively visualizing what you want.

Athletes do it all the time. They concentrate and picture themselves winning an event. Even before it happens, they picture in great detail all the steps they will take to win. The technique is also used in education, psychotherapy, stress management, and self-healing for cancer and other diseases. There's nothing new or unusual about it. It is something everyone can use.

Why should I do creative visualization?

Visualization teaches you how you can contribute positively to your life. It teaches you to go within yourself and discover the choices available to you and to choose what's best. Creative visualization is about trusting yourself and learning that you do have the power within yourself to make things work for you.

If you practice regularly, visualization skills will—

◆ Help you develop self-confidence.
◆ Improve your relationships.
◆ Help you relax and enjoy pregnancy and life.
◆ Promote relaxation of your body and mind.
◆ Help you make better birth plans.
◆ Help you think more positively about yourself.

◆ Reduce your fear of pregnancy and childbirth.
◆ Reduce your pain in labor.
◆ Help you bond with your baby before she or he is born.
◆ Reduce the likelihood of your having postpartum blues.

Visualization can be used to create anything positive you desire. It is something you can use when you like—not just during pregnancy, labor, and birth. If you consistently practice during pregnancy, you will see how you can use it for other things. You should practice every day.

There is one rule: What you visualize must always be positive and good for you.

For the Labor Companion

Visualization skills can be practiced by the labor companion also. Regular practice will help develop the labor companion's confidence in the birth process and his or her ability to give effective labor support.

How to Visualize

First, find a quiet place where you won't be interrupted. You may sit or lie down. The most important thing is that you get comfortable.

Find someone who can read the Visualization Practice Sheet to you, or tape it yourself with soft music in the background. It is only a guide. You can even make up your own. Participate in whatever way is most helpful to you. There is no right or wrong way. Some people have a hard time seeing pictures in their head, but they can sense them in other ways.

Keep a journal of your visualization practices. After each practice session, write down what you visualized and how you felt about it. Your visualization skills will improve every time you practice.

Visualization Practice Sheet

"Your Special Place"

Close your eyes and, when you are ready, begin to relax.

♦

Imagine every muscle in your body beginning to relax... starting from your toes and moving up to the tip of your scalp. Feel all of the stress and discomfort just lifting off of your body and disappearing.

♦

Count down slowly from 10 to 1... feeling yourself more and more relaxed and peaceful with each slow count.

♦

Breathe in deeply and slowly from way inside your belly. Imagine a golden beam of light filling your body with each breath. See the light surrounding your body and your baby's... protecting each of you with its warm, healing energy.

♦

When you begin to feel really relaxed, take a journey... to a very special place inside your mind. Imagine yourself in a beautiful natural environment. It can be real or imagined. Any place you like... a lush mountaintop... a splashing waterfall... a sunny beach... a tropical garden.... It can be anywhere in the universe, as long as it feels beautiful, comfortable, and peaceful.

♦

This is your secret place... your sanctuary.... Nothing bad can happen here. You are protected... safe... peaceful....

♦

Next, explore your place. Notice your surroundings. Breathe in the smells. Listen to the sounds....

♦

Now take some time to walk very slowly through this special place. Feel what it feels like to be in this place of wonder.

♦

Do anything you want to make this place more like home for you. You may build a cozy cabin... a steepled castle... put up a swaying hammock... add tropical singing birds... anything to make this place a more relaxing, peaceful sanctuary.

♦

After you have designed it, find a comfortable spot to sit in it. Look at what surrounds you. Study the magnificence and know that this is your special place. Nothing can harm you. Only good things happen here. You designed this beautiful place. If any bad thoughts come in, just tell them to go away. This is your place... your inner sanctuary. You may come here to relax and be free from worry any time. You may even change it to make it more beautiful every time you come.

♦

Notice how good you feel! How healthy and wonderful! Now begin to think of something good you would like to happen in your life. A healthy pregnancy... a loving relationship... a better job... any wish... anything that will make you happy... anything that will take away your worries and stress.

♦

(Continued)

Visualization Practice Sheet

Now pick one wish and focus on how you would feel if you were granted your wish. You can bring anyone or anything into your place that will help make your wish come true. Remember that you are still in your special place and that all wishes can be granted.

◆

What do you see and feel? Who is helping you? How are they making you feel so good? What are they saying to you?

◆

What has happened to make your wish come true? Let any image come in and play.

◆

Imagine how your life would be with this wish coming true. Imagine how life would be without your worries. Picture yourself already in this situation. Imagine how good you feel inside… how beautiful… how comfortable… how happy. Feel the laughter… the joy… the peace of heart. Keep the golden rays of light around your body and feel their radiance warm you like magic.

◆

Enjoy these feelings. Thank everyone and everything in your special place for being there for you to enjoy. Thank them for their help. And thank yourself for creating this beautiful sanctuary.

◆

Take a last look around at your special place. Remember its details. Tell it that you'll be back very soon.

◆

Slowly let it go and begin your journey back. Counting from 1 to 10, concentrate on each and every slow… deep… relaxing breath. Feel the lightness in your body. Feel the golden rays penetrating throughout, energizing your body. At the count of 10, very s–l–o–w–l–y open your eyes. Stay   still for a few moments before getting up…   *(End of visualization)*

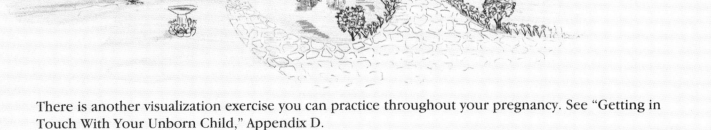

There is another visualization exercise you can practice throughout your pregnancy. See "Getting in Touch With Your Unborn Child," Appendix D.

The Next Step

Now that you have completed the first module, you may want to take some time to think about how you can use this information in your everyday life. Below is a list of activities to help you fully experience what you have learned:

- Review the glossary so you can understand and talk with your health care provider.
- Keep notes on how you feel (mentally and physically) and notice the changes you are experiencing.
- Watch what you eat and drink. Try to eat the best things for you and your baby.
- Avoid harmful substances. Make responsible decisions for yourself and your baby.
- Keep exercising. If you aren't already, think about the most fun exercise you can do that will benefit your body.
- Practice relaxation and visualization. You will be amazed at how well they work.
- Be careful. You can prevent injuries to yourself and your baby.
- Plan ahead for your baby. Review the appendixes for ideas.
- Enjoy yourself as much as possible. This is a new, wonderful time in your life.

Module II
Labor and Birth

Can it be? By now you are probably past the halfway mark of pregnancy and are thinking about labor and birth. It's important to learn all that you can now about what to expect and how you can prepare for the birth of your baby. Module II discusses labor and birth in detail.

Chapter 5 provides basic information on what to expect during labor, including how to know if you are in labor. Chapter 6 discusses skills for coping with labor and gives you hints on how to practice them. Chapter 7 talks about choices, variations, and complications in labor.

5 *Labor and You*

In this chapter, you will learn—
- Terms used in labor.
- How to know when you are in labor.
- How to time contractions.
- What to expect during different stages of labor.
- What causes pain in labor.

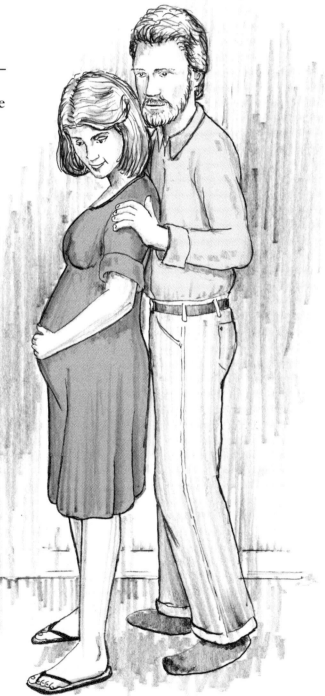

You've taken care of yourself during pregnancy, done all the right things, carried a growing baby for nine months, and now you are probably thinking, "I can't wait for this baby to be born!" For most women, the major question at the end of pregnancy is "What will labor **really** be like?" You may wonder how you will know when to go to the hospital, how to time contractions, and what will actually happen to your body during labor. In this chapter you will learn the answers to these questions and more. During class you will also practice techniques for coping with labor.

If you've never had a baby, your expectations of labor probably consist of what you've been told. Take a few minutes to think about what you've heard from your mother, from friends, from relatives, from others. If you've already had a baby, think about how it felt. Spend a few minutes writing down your thoughts below and have your labor companion write down his or her thoughts also. Then you can discuss what you already know and what you want and need to learn.

What I've heard about labor or what I've experienced in labor

_____

_____

_____

_____

_____

_____

_____

_____

_____

_____

_____

_____

What Is Labor?

Labor is the process by which your baby is born. Your uterus contracts, your cervix opens, and your baby travels from the uterus, through the pelvis, and then through the birth canal to the outside world. To understand labor, it is helpful to know the common terms used to describe its various phases. Knowing the terms will help you to discuss labor with your health care provider and to understand your progress during labor. Some of these terms are defined below:

◆ **Engagement (Fig. 14)** Near the end of your pregnancy, the baby moves deeper into your pelvis. This is called engagement. People may say your baby has "dropped" or "lightening" has occurred. You may feel more pressure on your bladder and have to go to the bathroom more often, but you will probably be able to breathe more easily. Engagement can happen as early as four weeks before your due date. If you've had a baby before, it might not happen until labor begins.

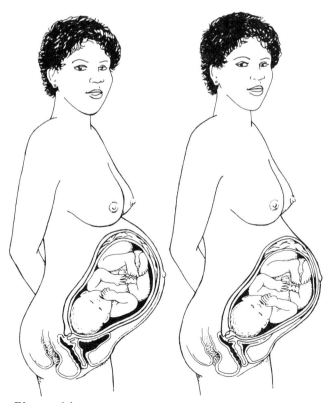

Figure 14

◆ **Effacement and dilatation *(Fig. 15)*** Your cervix (the neck or bottom part of your uterus) must thin out and open during labor. The thinning out is called effacement. Effacement is measured in percentages: 0 to 100 percent. Your cervix may begin to efface in the last weeks of your pregnancy, even before you are in labor.

Your cervix must open to 10 centimeters (about 4 inches) for the baby's head to pass through. This is called dilatation. This opening happens gradually, over a period of hours during labor. Sometimes the cervix begins to open (one to two centimeters) before labor begins. Your health care provider can check the progress of your labor by doing a vaginal exam to see how many centimeters you are dilated.

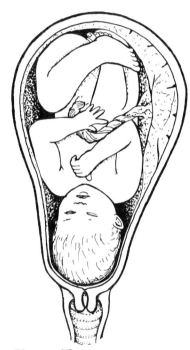 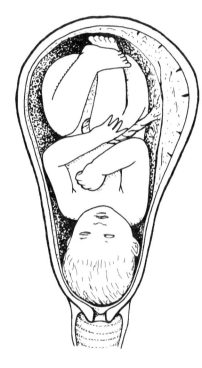 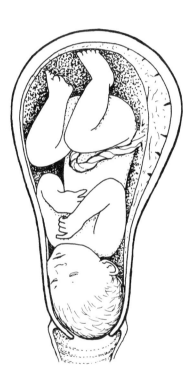

Figure 15

Labor and You

◆ **Presentation**—By the end of labor, about 95 percent of babies are positioned so the head will be born first. This is called a vertex or cephalic presentation *(Fig. 16)*. When a baby's position has the buttocks or legs coming first, it is called a breech

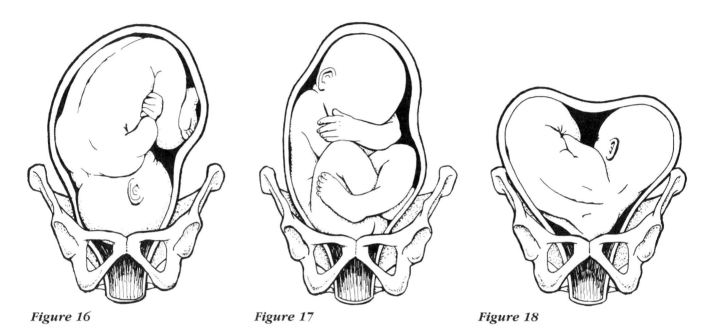

Figure 16   *Figure 17*   *Figure 18*

presentation *(Fig. 17)*. A transverse presentation occurs when a baby is lying across the uterus *(Fig. 18)*. Transverse and breech presentations may require that the mother have a cesarean birth to deliver the baby safely.

◆ **Station *(Fig. 19)*** To find out how far down into your pelvis the baby's head has traveled, your health care provider will measure the head's distance from an imaginary line in the middle of your pelvis. This measurement is called the station. If the baby's head is level with this line, it is at 0 station. If the head is above the line, it is at –1, –2, –3, or –4 station; if the head is below the line, it is at +1, +2, +3, or +4 station. (The measurements are in centimeters.) The head is engaged when it is at 0 station.

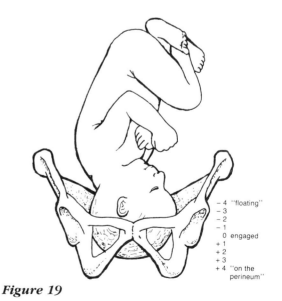

Figure 19

How Will I Know I'm in Labor?

In the last weeks of pregnancy, you wait and wonder when the baby will come. You begin to look for signs that labor is about to begin. Some of the signs that may indicate that labor will begin in a few days are—

◆ **Back pain**—Usually this is lower back pain that may come and go or be constant and become more intense over time.

◆ **Diarrhea**—Often a woman has loose stools for a day or two prior to labor.

◆ **Energy spurt/nesting instinct**—A woman may feel that she wants to scrub floors, paint the whole house, clean the closet, etc. She must be careful not to exhaust herself before labor begins.

◆ **Increased Braxton Hicks contractions**— These are painless and/or short contractions that may be regular or irregular, usually lasting for less than 30 seconds.

Some of the signs that labor may begin soon or has begun are—

◆ **Bloody show**—This pink or light red, thick discharge from the vagina is the mucous plug that falls from the cervix as it begins to dilate. It may appear a day or more before labor begins. If you have any bright red bleeding, call your health care provider or clinic at once.

◆ **Breaking the bag of waters** (rupture of membranes)—When the bag of waters breaks, the fluid can flow from the vagina in a sudden gush or in a trickle. When this happens, some women think they have lost control of their bladder. If your bag of waters breaks, or even if you **think** it might have broken but are not sure, call your health care provider or go to the hospital. Your bag of waters may break before you have any contractions or during contractions, or it might not break until very late in your labor.

If your bag of waters breaks before you get to the hospital, be sure to notice what color the fluid is or if there is any odor. Usually the fluid is clear or milky and has a mild odor. If it is greenish, yellowish, or dark, be sure to tell your health care provider when you call; this means the baby has had a bowel movement (has passed meconium) inside the amniotic sac. This is sometimes a sign that the baby is in fetal distress. If there is a foul odor, it may mean that you have an infection.

◆ **Contractions**—Contractions are the tightening of the muscles of the uterus. They usually begin mildly and get stronger, longer, and closer together as labor progresses. You may feel them in your back and then moving around to the front, low on the abdomen.

◆ **Dilatation of the cervix**—This is the opening up of your cervix. It is a sure sign of labor and can only be determined by a pelvic examination.

Note: You should have the Labor Telephone List (Appendix E) handy when you begin labor. Tear it out, fill in the blanks, and keep it by your telephone.

How Do Contractions Feel?

A contraction is like a wave: It begins gently, rises to a peak of intensity, and then drops off. Then there's a break before the next one begins. Here are some descriptions of what contractions feel like:

◆ "They felt like strong menstrual cramps at first."

◆ "I thought I had bad gas."

◆ "I felt everything in my back—like a bad backache that came and went."

◆ "Contractions felt like a pulling and stretching sensation—very strong."

◆ "They were very difficult near the end. I felt like the pain never stopped."

Note: If you begin to have regular contractions (more than four in one hour) before 37 weeks of pregnancy, call your health care provider or go to the hospital. You may be in premature labor.

How Do I Time My Contractions?

You and your labor companion should know how to time contractions. When your labor begins, your health care provider will ask you how long each contraction lasts and how much time there is between contractions. This information tells your health care provider how your labor is progressing. It also helps you to know when to call your health care provider and when to go to the hospital. Following is the correct procedure for timing your contractions—

◆ Have handy a pen or a pencil, paper, and a stopwatch or a clock with a second hand.

◆ Write down the time when a contraction begins. Then write down the time when that contraction ends. This will give you the length (duration) of each contraction. *(See Figure 20.)*

    Note the amount of time between the beginning of one contraction and the beginning of the next one. This is the frequency (interval) of contractions. For example, if one contraction begins at 7:30 and the next one begins at 7:37, the contractions are seven minutes apart.

◆ You do not have to time every contraction. Time four or five contractions, then stop for a while. Begin to time them again in an hour or so or if the rate or rhythm of the contractions seems to be changing or if there are other signs of labor.

◆ Call your health care provider when your contractions are five minutes apart for a first baby and 10 minutes apart if you've had other children or when your health care provider tells you to call.

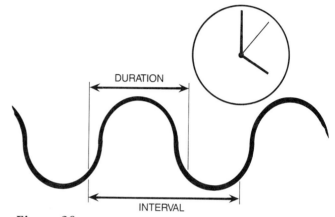

Figure 20

False Labor

Sometimes Braxton Hicks contractions, which occur throughout pregnancy, get very strong near the end of pregnancy and are very uncomfortable. Many women confuse these contractions with true labor contractions. This is what is known as prelabor or false labor. Strong Braxton Hicks contractions may occur for several days or weeks before labor begins. It can be very frustrating to go to the hospital because you think you are in labor, only to be sent home because you are not. The signs below can sometimes help you to tell the difference between true labor and false labor.

True Labor	False Labor
Contractions are usually regular.	Contractions are usually irregular.
Contractions get longer over time.	Contractions are short and don't get longer.
Contractions become more painful.	Contractions do not usually become very painful.
Contractions may intensify if you walk and they will not go away.	Contractions may stop if you get up and walk.
Bloody show may be present.	Bloody show is not present.
Your cervix dilates. (Determined by pelvic exam.)	Your cervix does not dilate. (Determined by pelvic exam.)

Stages of Labor

Labor has four distinct stages. During each stage, specific changes take place that require different adjustments by the laboring woman. The length and intensity of each stage varies from labor to labor, but every labor goes through each stage.

Stage I
Stage I covers the period from the first labor contraction until the cervix is 10 centimeters dilated. Stage I has three phases:
◆ Early labor—0 to 3 centimeters of dilatation.
◆ Active labor—4 to 7 centimeters of dilatation.
◆ Transition—8 to 10 centimeters of dilatation.

Stage II
Stage II begins when the woman reaches full dilatation (10 centimeters). It ends with the birth of the baby (the pushing stage).

Stage III
Stage III covers the period from the birth of the baby until the delivery of the placenta.

Stage IV
Stage IV includes the first hour or so of recovery and stabilization after delivery.

See the Labor Guide on pages 72–74 for information on what occurs during each stage, how you may feel, and how to cope.

The Baby's Journey

The baby's passage out of the uterus and through the vagina during the second stage of labor is not a straight one. Not only does the baby have to pass through the uterus and birth canal, he or she also must pass through the pelvis. *Figures 21–24* show how most babies turn during this journey. Usually the baby begins labor in a position facing the mother's side *(Fig. 21)*, then turns to face the mother's back *(Figs. 22a and b)*. The baby's head has to extend to pass under the pubic bone *(Fig. 23)* and then turns to the side for the birth of the shoulders *(Fig. 24)*.

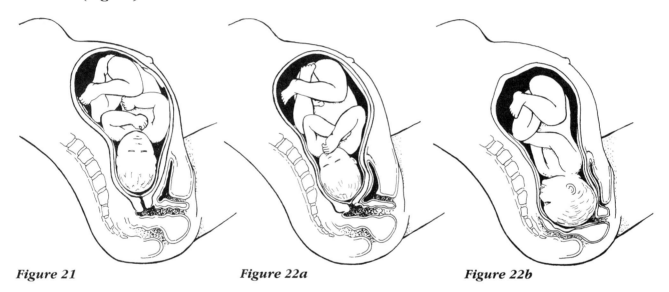

Figure 21   *Figure 22a*   *Figure 22b*

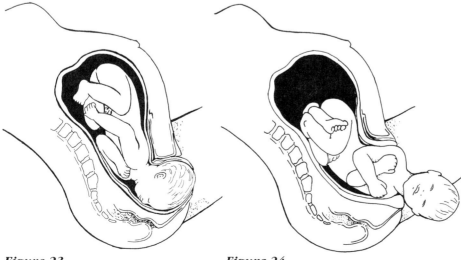

Figure 23   *Figure 24*

Discomfort and Pain in Labor

When asked what they worry about most concerning labor and delivery, most women say "the pain." Pain in labor ranges from very mild discomfort (not even as bad as cramps) to very intense sensations. Most women experience something in between. One of the purposes of this course is to teach you to cope with the discomforts and pain of labor.

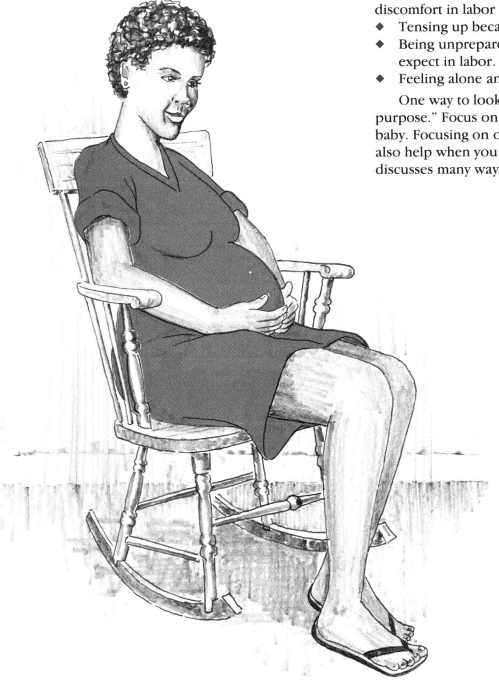

There are several physical causes of pain in labor:

◆ The stretching of the cervix and pressure of the baby on nerves and other body structures during labor.
◆ The feelings of pressure of the baby and stretching of the vagina as the baby moves down and out during the second stage of labor.
◆ Possible temporary lack of oxygen to the uterus as it contracts.

Other factors that may increase pain and discomfort in labor include—

◆ Tensing up because you are afraid of labor.
◆ Being unprepared and not knowing what to expect in labor.
◆ Feeling alone and unsupported.

One way to look at labor is as "pain with a purpose." Focus on the end result—a beautiful baby. Focusing on one contraction at a time will also help when you are in labor. Chapter 6 discusses many ways for coping with labor.

Labor Guide

This guide shows what happens to you physically during each stage of labor. It also shows various reactions experienced by women in labor and suggested activities for the woman and her labor companion. Use this guide as you plan for labor and birth. You may want to take it to the hospital with you to remind you of things to do during each stage.

Stage of Labor	What Happens	Possible Reactions	Suggested Activities for the Laboring Woman	Suggested Activities for the Labor Companion
Stage I **Phase 1:** Early Labor (Usually lasts 6–12 hours)	Cervix dilates 0–3 centimeters. Effacement begins or continues. Mucous plug may be lost. Bag of waters may break. Contractions are mild, 5–20 minutes apart, 30–40 seconds long.	Excited, happy, ready to rush to hospital and have the baby. Anxious.	Walk. Rest or sleep if labor begins during the night. Drink clear fluids. Use breathing and relaxation if needed. Finish packing.	Encourage comfort and relaxation and warm showers. Have her alternate walking and resting. Help time contractions and notify health care provider as appropriate. Encourage her to drink clear liquids. Discuss coping skills for use later in labor.
Phase 2: Active Labor (Usually lasts 2–6 hours)	Cervix dilates 4–7 centimeters. Effacement completed. Contractions are 3–6 minutes apart, 40–60 seconds long. Increased bloody show. Bag of waters may break.	Serious, more concentrated on the labor. Does not like outside distractions. Focused on self.	Anticipate and work with contractions. Use relaxation and breathing techniques as needed. Keep bladder empty. Walk. Change positions frequently.	Vary your efforts to keep her comfortable. Suggest position changes. Remind her to empty her bladder. Use massage, touch. Offer ice chips. Help her communicate needs and wishes to care givers.

Stage of Labor	What Happens	Possible Reactions	Suggested Activities for the Laboring Woman	Suggested Activities for the Labor Companion
Phase 3: Transition (Can last from a few minutes to several hours)	Cervix dilates 7–10 centimeters. Contractions are 2–3 minutes apart, 50–90 seconds long.	Feelings more intense. Needs more support. May be drowsy, forgetful, irrational. Nausea, hiccups. May have pressure on rectum. May feel discouraged, irritable. May sleep between contractions. May have leg cramps. May tremble. May feel a strong urge to push.	Take one contraction at a time. Tell someone if you have the urge to push. More concentrated attention to relaxation and breathing techniques may be needed.	Increase your help. Don't leave her alone during this time. May need to breathe with her through contractions. Stay calm, firm, confident. Give lots of encouragement. Be alert for signs of pushing. Notify care givers if she wants to push.
Stage II Pushing (Usually lasts 15 minutes to 3 hours)	Baby begins to pass out of the uterus and goes through the birth canal assisted by pushing efforts of mother. Contractions are 2–5 minutes apart, 45–60 seconds long.	May have new burst of energy. Excited. Contractions may be felt as less painful or more painful. Relieved to be able to push.	Push as directed. Relax the perineum. Be prepared to pant as the head is born. Continue to relax between contractions. Stay in upright position if possible. Change positions if labor is not progressing.	Help her to find a comfortable position for pushing. Encourage her efforts. Promote relaxation between contractions. Make her comfortable.

Labor Guide

Stage of Labor	What Happens	Possible Reactions	Suggested Activities for the Laboring Woman	Suggested Activities for the Labor Companion
Stage III Delivery of Placenta (Usually lasts 15–30 minutes)	Placenta delivered after the baby is born.	Happy and tired. May wish to see and hold baby. May feel hot or cold. Shaking.	Push as directed for delivery of placenta. Hold baby. Let care givers know your wishes; don't wait to be asked.	Share your feelings Hold the baby. Help mother communicate wishes to care givers.
Stage IV Recovery (Usually lasts 1–2 hours)	Period of stabilization after birth. Uterus begins to contract.	May have after-pains from contractions of uterus, vaginal bleeding, shaking, or chills. Care giver or mother may massage uterus. May feel elated, excited, want to hold and touch baby. May be laughing and crying. May feel exhausted.	Have contact with baby if possible. If you will breastfeed, begin soon after delivery. Keep warm. Enjoy the sense of accomplishment and relief.	Spend time with baby if possible. Cuddle, caress, and talk to him or her. Enjoy the sense of accomplishment and relief.

6 Coping With Labor

In this chapter, you will learn—
◆ Ways to prepare for your hospital stay.
◆ The importance of your labor companion and what he or she needs to know to help you.
◆ Different skills for coping with labor.
◆ Information on various medications that are sometimes used in labor.

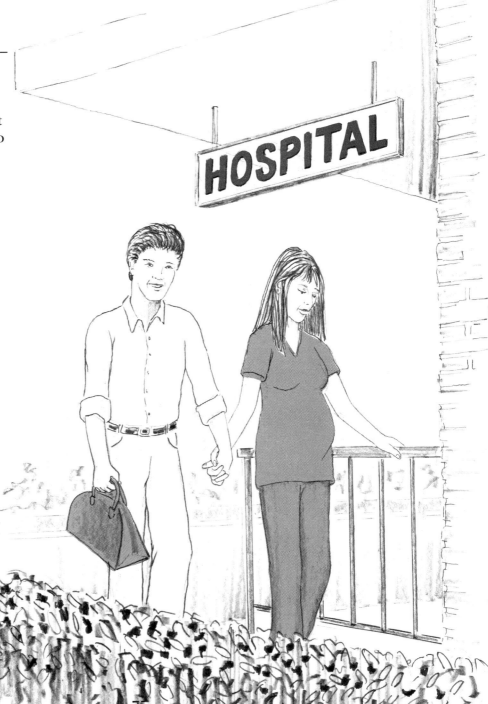

Knowing what to expect during labor and birth will help you become more confident about your pregnancy. Attending classes, reading, and discussing your concerns with your health care provider and labor companion are ways to help you feel more secure. Practicing what you already know, such as relaxation and visualization, can also be useful.

Labor is a team effort. You, your labor companion, your health care provider, and other health care personnel will be working together during your labor for the birth of your baby. There are many ways that you and your support team can work together to make your labor more enjoyable and more comfortable.

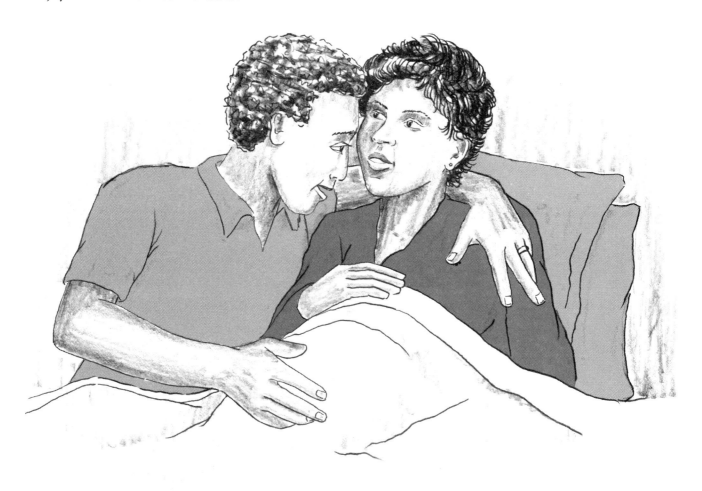

Preparing for Your Hospital Stay

One of the easiest things you can do to have things run smoothly is to be prepared. Use the checklist below as a guide for things you can take care of in advance. Check off each task as you complete it.

_____ Preregister at the hospital.

_____ Check your insurance coverage if you have insurance.

_____ Make a practice run to the hospital with your labor companion.

_____ Know how to get to the hospital if your labor companion can't drive you.

_____ Know which entrance of the hospital to use during the day and which to use at night.

_____ Arrange child care for other children in your home.

_____ Put towels in the car in case your water breaks while you are in the car.

_____ Pack your "labor room bag."

_____ Pack your suitcase for the postpartum stay.

_____ Prepare and freeze meals for your first days at home.

_____ Plan how to get help at home.

_____ Tell your health care provider what you want to happen during labor and after.

Labor Room Bag

Following is a list of items you may want to use while you are in labor. Go over this list and choose the things you think would be helpful or useful. Add your own ideas of what would help make you feel comfortable.

- Something you like to look at that you can use during relaxation and breathing. This could be a picture of a beautiful place, a flower, a loved one, or anything else.
- Lip moisturizer or petroleum jelly for dry lips.
- Lotion, cornstarch, or baby powder for massage.
- Games or cards to fill the time during early labor.
- Tapes of your favorite music and a tape player or a radio. Check with your hospital to see if you need battery-powered equipment.
- Meal for your labor companion. Pack food that won't spoil and that doesn't have a strong odor.
- Camera and film.
- Notebook and pencil.
- Phone numbers and enough change for the person who will make those first phone calls.
- Pillows to use for comfort in labor. Use your most colorful pillow cases so that your pillows don't get mixed in with the hospital supply.
- Something nice to hold, like a favorite stone, a stuffed animal, or a piece of soft cloth.
- _slippers / socks (padded)_
- _bathrobe_
- _nursing bra_
  toothbrush   shampoo/conditioner
  toothpaste   deodorant

The Importance of Support

1-2 baby outfits/going home outfit/blanket

One of the most important gifts a woman can receive during labor is support from another person. Whether this is her husband, her mother, her friend, a nurse, or anyone else does not matter. The only important things are that the laboring woman can trust this person and

list of insurance # + info.
car seat

work with him or her in labor and that this person understands what is helpful to her. Studies have shown that women who have support during labor have shorter labors and fewer complications. When asked what helped them the most during labor, most women say it was the support they received from their labor companion.

It is very important that your labor companion know the best ways to help you. If you both attend a course such as this one and practice regularly together, you will begin to work as a team in preparing for labor. Some labor companions play a very active role during labor; others provide support just by their presence. It is up to the two of you to decide how you can best work together.

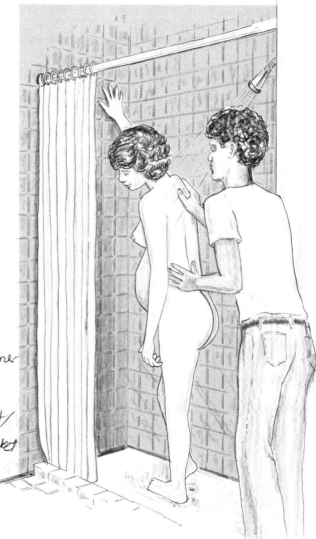

For the Labor Companion

Your role as a labor companion is very important. You are the expectant mother's guide and her best friend at this time. From the very beginning you have to be there for her. She needs you to comfort, reassure, and encourage her through the whole labor process. As a labor companion, you can help her cope with labor and also with the hospital environment. Some of the concerns that labor companions often have are discussed below.

"I'm worried I will feel totally helpless when she's in labor and not be able to help out at all. What can I really do?"

Many women say that just having a loved one present with them is the best support. In addition, there **are** many ways that you can help her during labor. For example, you can help her breathe during the more difficult contractions, massage her sore back, and offer her ice chips. You can also help her visualize the baby being born. Most important, you can give her encouragement and tell her she is doing a great job.

"How can I prepare for this job?"

There are many ways for you to prepare for the job of labor companion. You should—
◆ Meet the health care provider ahead of time, if possible. Doing this will help you feel like part of the team when labor begins.
◆ Take childbirth classes.
◆ Tour the hospital.
◆ Practice breathing, relaxation, and visualization with the expectant mother.
◆ Discuss with the expectant mother what is

important to her during labor and birth. It may be such things as avoiding medication, if possible; using the birthing room; or spending time with the baby after birth. Have a clear understanding of what she wants and does not want.

"I don't think I can stand to see her in pain."

It is sometimes difficult to watch someone you care about in pain. Usually, by working together before the labor and in early labor, you will have an idea of what the laboring woman needs and wants during the different stages of labor. Having this information can help you work together to decrease pain. If you feel insecure at any time, a care giver is always near to help you remember some coping techniques. **You may be tempted to ask for pain medication for the laboring woman, but she is the one who should make the decision about taking medication.** Remind her to use her favorite relaxation, visualization, or breathing skills. Massage her shoulders, sing to her, help keep up her spirits. During labor, she may cry, scream, or yell at you. Try to be patient, kind, and understanding, and know that she will get through labor more easily with your help.

"How much blood will there be?"

There is much less blood involved than you probably imagine. Also, most labor companions are working too hard to notice anyway.

"What if I faint?"

A prepared labor companion rarely faints, but if you do feel faint, ask for help. The nursing staff is there to assist both of you.

Skills for Coping With Labor

There are many ways you can cope with labor. In Chapter 4, you practiced progressive relaxation and visualization. You may be familiar already with some of the others listed below. In this section, you will learn more about the skills that can make your labor easier and possibly more enjoyable. They are—
◆ Relaxation.
◆ Visualization.
◆ Breathing.
◆ Focusing.
◆ Positioning.

Relaxation

Women differ in what helps them to relax with their contractions. Being able to relax in labor can help the uterus do the work of contracting without interference. There are many different types of relaxation skills used for labor. Here you will practice progressive relaxation and touch relaxation. Also, briefly discussed are meditation as a form of relaxation and music as a way to enhance relaxation.

It is important that you try different methods so you can decide which works best for you.

Progressive Relaxation

You already know about progressive relaxation, which was discussed and practiced in Chapter 4. Practice this method with your labor companion.

Touch Relaxation

Relaxation in response to touch can be very effective during labor. You and your labor companion should become familiar with the techniques described on the next page.

Other Relaxation Methods

There are other personal things you can do to relax. **Meditation** is one of the oldest methods of relaxing. It can be done in almost the same way you do visualization (see Chapter 4). To meditate, you usually need to find a very quiet, comfortable place to sit. In labor, you might not have this luxury. However, you can still meditate by reaching into yourself and focusing on your breathing and your own inner thoughts. Generally, meditation is done alone without guidance from someone else. If you wish to be alone with your thoughts, explain this desire to your labor companion. Just having that person near may be all the comfort you need while you meditate.

Music is one of the most relaxing tools available. Pick out your favorite music and listen to it. Notice how it makes you feel. You may use music along with any form of relaxation or visualization. Music can also be used as a focal point for your attention. Whatever method of relaxation you use, try to practice it on a regular basis.

Visualization

Creative visualization was discussed and practiced in Chapter 4. Creative visualization in labor can be used to increase relaxation and decrease pain. Some of the benefits of visualization during labor are that it—

◆ Helps you to relax.
◆ Prevents you from getting too tired.
◆ Makes labor less painful.
◆ Helps increase oxygen to both you and the baby.
◆ Reduces fear.
◆ Helps reduce the length of labor.
◆ Helps create a positive birth experience.

There are a number of visualization exercises you can do. Three easy ones are—

◆ **Special place**—The special place visualization is very good to use in the birthing setting because it can make you feel totally comfortable even though you are in an unfamiliar place. Practice this exercise as suggested on page 57. Remember that using music with it will make it even more pleasant.

◆ **Wave**—Imagine your contractions as waves. Imagine that you are a surfer on these waves. With each contraction you are riding smoothly through to the next set of waves. Imagine at the peak of each contraction that you have successfully reached the top of a wave. When each wave comes, you become more confident and secure. You begin to see yourself as an accomplished surfer, fully in control, always able to pull yourself through.

◆ **Flower**—Imagine the baby coming down through your birth canal. Imagine your cervix opening up like the petals of a beautiful flower. Picture the flower and its beauty as specifically as you can. Make it any color and any shape. Watch each petal open gradually. As the flower opens, your baby is moving through the birth canal. Talk to your baby as you practice this exercise.

Note: Practice the flower visualization only when you are in labor.

Touch Relaxation Practice Sheet

Touch relaxation involves having your labor companion touch or massage various parts of your body. Sometimes it is easier to relax with a touch than by just being told to relax. When you practice touch relaxation, have your labor companion experiment with different kinds of touch. Let him or her know what feels best—a light touch, firm stroking along your arms and legs, a firm neck and shoulder massage, or any other type of touch. Practice the following relaxation skills with your labor companion.

Relax Your Head

- Raise your eyebrows and wrinkle your forehead.
- Have your labor companion stroke your forehead, beginning in the middle and working out to the temples.
- Tense your scalp.
- Have your labor companion massage your scalp with his or her fingertips.

Relax Your Neck

- Tense your neck.
- Have your labor companion touch your shoulders firmly.
  or
- Tense your neck.
- Have your labor companion massage your shoulders.

Relax Your Arms

- With your right arm, make a fist and tighten the entire arm.
- Have your labor companion stroke down the arm from the shoulder to the fingertips.
- Have your labor companion massage your hand.
- Repeat with the left arm.

Relax Your Lower Back

- Lie on your side.
- Arch your lower back.
- Have your labor companion massage your lower back, beginning in the center and moving outward.
  or
- Lie on your side.
- Arch your lower back.
- Have your labor companion stroke down your back from the shoulders to the buttocks on either side of your spine.

Relax Your Lower Legs

- Lie on your back.
- Tighten the muscles of both of your legs, pointing your toes toward your nose.
- Have your labor companion stroke down the sides of your legs from the hip to the foot.
- Have your labor companion massage your feet.

Note: Be sure not to massage or use deep pressure around the calves, because pregnant women are more likely to develop blood clots that could be dislodged.

Attention: Labor Companion

Look carefully at the pregnant woman. Try to see where she holds her tension. Some women may clench their fists, some may draw up their shoulders, others may clamp their jaws together. If you can see when she is tense, help her to relax.

A tense muscle is tight and a relaxed muscle is soft. To check her arms or legs for tension, lift them gently. If they are relaxed, they will be heavy and loose and she won't be helping you to lift them. If they are tense, they will be stiff and she will probably help you lift them.

If she is tense, tell her in your own words to "let go," "release," and "relax," and use some of the touch relaxation skills you have learned. Some techniques will work better for her than others, and some will work better at different times during labor.

Once you have worked together as a team for a while, you might try this exercise. As she tightens her right arm, check to see if her left arm is relaxed. Do the same for her legs. As you get better at this, you can play a game of "hide and seek"—she tenses a part of her body and you guess which part is tensed and help her to relax it.

Breathing Instruction and Practice

Using special breathing techniques during labor can help you in several ways. Slow, deep breathing often aids muscle relaxation. It can also offer a distraction from the strong contractions you will have during labor. Slow, deep, relaxed breathing can provide needed oxygen to you and the baby during labor. Some women find that simple deep breathing during labor is all they need; others need more complex patterns to help them out. As with any coping technique, some will work better for you than others. Below are descriptions of six breathing techniques starting with the simplest, and going through the types used in each stage of labor and delivery. For some of the exercises, you will need a stopwatch or a clock with a second hand.

As you practice, you will notice that fast breathing is more tiring than slow breathing. Therefore use fast breathing only if it helps you to cope with contractions better. In labor, begin by breathing slowly and then speed your breathing to match the strength of the contraction. When the contraction begins to get less intense, begin to slow your breathing again. Always begin and end each practice contraction with a cleansing breath.

1. **Cleansing breath** is a deep breath in through your nose and out through your mouth. It acts as a signal to your body to relax and breathe. It also increases oxygen to your body and to the baby.

Practice the Cleansing Breath

- Take a deep breath in through your nose.
- Breathe out through your mouth as you relax completely.

---

2. **Slow breathing** is used in early labor and in active labor, although some women use it throughout their labor.

    Have your labor companion count how many breaths you normally take in one minute. (This is usually 12 to 20 breaths per minute.) For slow breathing, take about half that number of breaths each minute. You may want to breathe in through your nose and out through your mouth. If you have a stuffy nose, breathe only through your mouth.

    Practice several pretend 60-second contractions each day.

Practice Slow Breathing

- Get into a comfortable position. Contraction begins. Take a cleansing breath. Relax.
- Breathe in and out very slowly and steadily. In… out… . In… out… . In… out… . Keep your breathing steady and even. Continue for about 60 seconds. Contraction ends.
- Take a cleansing breath.
- Repeat several times.

---

3. **Modified paced breathing** is used in active labor and in transition if slow breathing is no longer effective. It is faster than normal breathing, up to twice the normal rate (24 to 40 breaths a minute). It is usually done in and out through the mouth. The breaths are light and done with little effort. Practice to find your own rate and rhythm, which will be different for each person.

    Practice several pretend 60-second to 90-second contractions each day.

Practice Modified Paced Breathing

- Get into a comfortable position. Contraction begins.
- Take a cleansing breath. Relax.
- Breathe lightly, with little effort, at 24 to 40 breaths per minute. Some women like to make sounds on the out-breath such as "Ha…Ha…Ha… ." Continue for 60 to 90 seconds. Contraction ends.
- Take a cleansing breath.
- Repeat several times.

---

4. **Patterned paced breathing** is used in active labor and in transition. The number of breaths per minute is the same as in modified paced breathing, but in patterned paced breathing you blow out forcefully every several breaths. Patterned breathing focuses your attention on counting and on varying the activity, which can be a help during active labor. Some women use a pattern of breaths and blows, for example, three breaths, blow, four breaths, blow, three breaths, blow. Others have their labor companion hold up fingers to indicate the number of breaths to give before blowing out.

Practice several pretend 60-second to 90-second contractions each day.

Practice Patterned Paced Breathing

♦ Get into a comfortable position. Contraction begins.
♦ Take a cleansing breath. Relax.
♦ Breath in and out, giving an outward blow every three to four breaths. Breathe lightly, with little effort. (While you are learning, work on finding your own rhythm and rate.) Contraction ends.
♦ Take a cleansing breath.
♦ Repeat several times.

---

5. **Breathing to avoid pushing** is used near the end of labor when you have the urge to push but must avoid pushing until the cervix is completely dilated.

Practice Breathing to Avoid Pushing

♦ Pant as you take small breaths in and out through your mouth or blow out with your lips pursed as if you were blowing out a birthday candle.

---

6. **Breathing for birth** is used when the cervix is completely dilated and you are helping to push the baby down the birth canal and out. (*Warning:* Do not actually push or bear down when you practice.)

Practice Breathing for Birth

*(When you are in labor, you will actually push. Do **not** push when you practice.)*

♦ Take two cleansing breaths.
♦ Get into a good position for pushing. Breathe in. Relax the perineum.
♦ Pretend you are giving a steady push for five to six seconds.
♦ Take a small breath.
♦ Pretend to push again.
♦ Repeat several times until the contraction is over.
♦ Take a cleansing breath. Relax.

Focusing

Concentrating hard on something—focusing—helps some women work with their contractions. The object, activity, or idea concentrated on is called a focal point. You can focus on something in the room or on something that you have brought with you. Some women focus on a flower, a stone, a favorite picture or photo, or another special thing. Other women find it helpful to hum or make other sounds during breathing. Still others count with their breathing or focus on a movement such as rocking. Some women find closing their eyes and focusing inward, as in meditation, to be helpful. Focusing can be used with any of the relaxation, visualization, breathing, or positioning techniques discussed in this chapter.

Practice focusing during pretend contractions.

Positioning

The position a laboring woman is in has a lot to do with how comfortable she is. Frequent changes of position during labor will help you be more comfortable and improve the efficiency and strength of your contractions. You should avoid lying flat on your back during labor because this position decreases the efficiency of your contractions, is uncomfortable, and can decrease blood flow to the baby.

During Labor

While you are in labor—

◆ Walking upright can increase the strength and efficiency of contractions *(Fig. 25)*.

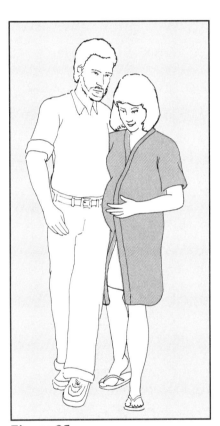

Figure 25

◆ Sitting up in a bed or a chair can be very comfortable *(Fig. 26)*.

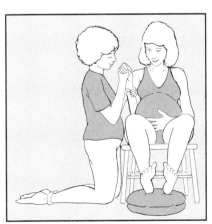

Figure 26

- A hands-and-knees position can ease back pain and abdominal discomfort *(Fig. 27)*.

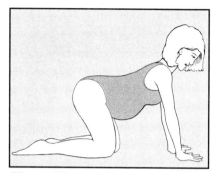

Figure 27

- Leaning against the back of a chair or the head of a bed with your head forward can help you relax your upper body *(Fig. 28)*.

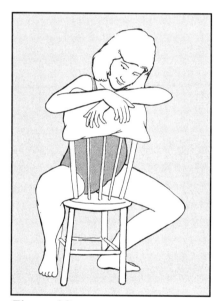

Figure 28

- Using your partner for support can make you more comfortable *(Fig. 29)*.

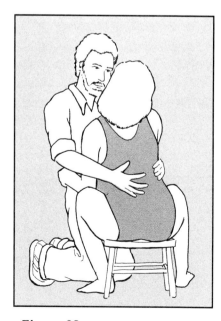

Figure 29

During Pushing and Birth

The positions you use for pushing will depend on many factors: the speed of your labor, your willingness and ability to move about (you may be hampered by a fetal monitor, an intravenous injection, epidural anesthesia, or a narrow bed), and your and the health care provider's preferences. As in labor, you should change positions during pushing, especially if you are pushing for a long time or the baby is moving down slowly.

While you are pushing and giving birth, remember that—

◆ Semisitting in bed, or using your labor companion for support, is a common position for pushing *(Fig. 30)*.

◆ If you must lie on your back, make sure you put pillows under your head and shoulders *(Fig. 31)*.

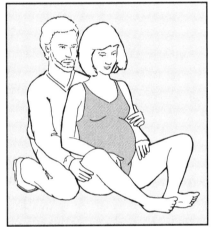

Figure 30

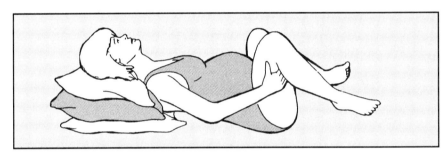

Figure 31

◆ A side-lying position with your partner holding and supporting your upper leg as you push is helpful *(Fig. 32)*.

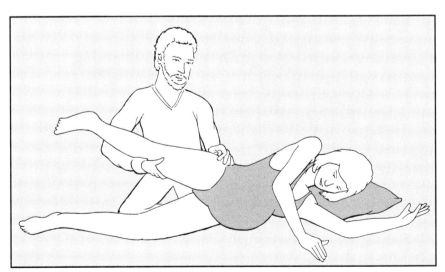

Figure 32

◆ Squatting can also assist the descent of the baby *(Fig. 33)*.

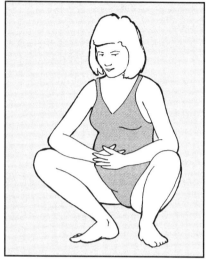

Figure 33

◆ The hands-and-knees position can make you more comfortable and assist in the descent of the baby *(Fig. 34)*.

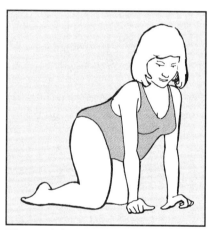

Figure 34

Medications During Labor

Sometimes, for medical reasons, women are given medication during labor. Sometimes women ask for medication to make them more comfortable. Medication requested by a woman in labor might or might not be given depending on the stage of labor and the condition of the baby.

It is important to understand what medications are available during labor and how each type works so that you can make an informed decision about having medication during your labor. Whether or not you use pain medication (except in emergency situations) is up to you. You should discuss medications with your health care provider before your labor begins. He or she can advise you about the types of medication used. All medication used for pain relief during labor may have some effect on the baby.

Questions About Medication

You should ask your health care provider the following questions:

- What medications do your patients usually receive? Why do they receive them? What are the side effects of these medications?
- What types of medications do you recommend for a difficult, painful, or prolonged delivery? For a cesarean?
- How can I avoid using pain medication if that is a goal for me?
- Other questions I have:

_____

_____

_____

Specific Medications

The medications used during labor and birth can be divided into three main groups:

- Systemic medications that enter the bloodstream and affect the whole body.
- Regional anesthesia, which produces numbness in a certain area of the body.
- General anesthesia, which causes unconsciousness in the mother.

The chart on pages 89–92 gives specific information on these medications.

Medications Used During Labor

Systemic Medications

Type of Drug	Names	When Used	Advantages	Disadvantages
Sedative	Seconal, Nembutal, Amytal, Phenobarbital (Given in a pill or an injection.)	Before active labor starts.	Allows woman to rest when she is exhausted.	Drowsiness in mother. If given shortly before the baby is born, the newborn is likely to have a decrease in alertness, sucking, and motor activity.
Tranquilizer	Valium, Vistaril, Phenergan, Sparine (Given in an injection or IV.)	Active labor.	Decreases anxiety. Enhances effect of narcotics so less narcotic medication can be used. Vistaril and Phenergan decrease nausea and vomiting.	If used alone, no pain relief for the mother. Valium can cause a decrease in alertness, sucking, and activity in the newborn.
Narcotic Analgesics	Demerol, Stadol, Nubain, Morphine (Given in an injection or IV.) *Nimorphan*	Active labor. Postpartum recovery from cesarean birth.	Effective pain relief. May improve mother's ability to use other coping techniques.	May cause drowsiness, confusion, nausea. Can make it difficult to concentrate on other coping techniques. Can slow labor if given early in labor. If administered too close to birth, can cause breathing problems for the newborn, as well as a decrease in alertness, sucking, and motor activity. Because of this, narcotics are usually not administered to laboring women in high dosages or late in labor.

Regional Anesthesia

Names	Type of Procedure	When Used	Advantages	Disadvantages
"Caine" drugs—Nesacaine, Xylocaine or Lidocaine, Marcaine or Bupivacaine, Carbocaine	Local anesthesia (Injected into the perineum to numb the area.)	At birth, for episiotomy and repair.	Quick and easy to administer. No known effects on the newborn.	Effective only in local area where it is administered.
	Pudendal block (Injected through the vagina into a ligament on either side of the vaginal wall.)	Second stage of labor. For forceps deliveries.	Pain relief.	May be ineffective in relieving pain.
	Paracervical block (Injected into either side of the cervix.)	Late in the first stage of labor.	Pain relief.	May be ineffective in relieving pain. Can cause decrease in fetal heart rate, so it is rarely used.
	Spinal or saddle block (Injected into the spinal canal.)	Forceps delivery. Cesarean birth.	Good pain relief.	Discomfort when being done. Loss of urge to push (forceps may be necessary). Possible spinal headache—like a severe migraine headache. May lower mother's blood pressure and decrease blood flow to the baby. This can be corrected or prevented with IV fluids or medication.

Regional Anesthesia

Names	Type of Procedure	When Used	Advantages	Disadvantages
	Caudal block (Injection outside the spinal canal near the base of the spine.)	Active labor. Forceps delivery. Cannot be used for a cesarean section.	Good pain relief. Can be readministered through catheter as needed. May be allowed to wear off in late labor so that mother can push more effectively.	Procedure is slightly uncomfortable (woman must be still for 5 to 10 minutes in awkward position). Sometimes pain relief is incomplete. Labor may slow; oxytocin may be used. May lower mother's blood pressure and decrease blood flow to the baby. This can be corrected with IV fluids or medications. Other interventions may include electronic fetal monitoring, bladder catheterization, and forceps delivery.

Regional Anesthesia

Names	Type of Procedure	When Used	Advantages	Disadvantages
	Epidural block (A tiny catheter inserted outside of the spinal canal in the middle of the back that remains in place throughout the delivery.) *(See Figure 35.)*	Active labor. Forceps delivery. Cesarean birth.	Good pain relief. Can be readministered through catheter as needed. Mother can be awake for delivery, even with cesarean. May be allowed to wear off in late labor so that mother can push more effectively.	Procedure is slightly uncomfortable (woman must be still for 5 to 10 minutes in awkward position). Sometimes pain relief is incomplete. Labor may slow; oxytocin may be used. May lower mother's blood pressure and decrease blood flow to the baby. This can be corrected with IV fluids or medications. Other interventions may include electronic fetal monitoring, bladder catheterization, and forceps delivery.

Figure 35

General Anesthesia

Names	Type of Procedure	When Used	Advantages	Disadvantages
Ethrane, nitrous oxide, Penthrane, Trilene	Administered through breathing tube with oxygen.	Cesarean birth.	Complete pain relief and rest.	Mother is unconscious. May inhale own vomit, resulting in breathing problems and pneumonia. May cause respiratory and heart rate problems or decreased alertness in newborn.

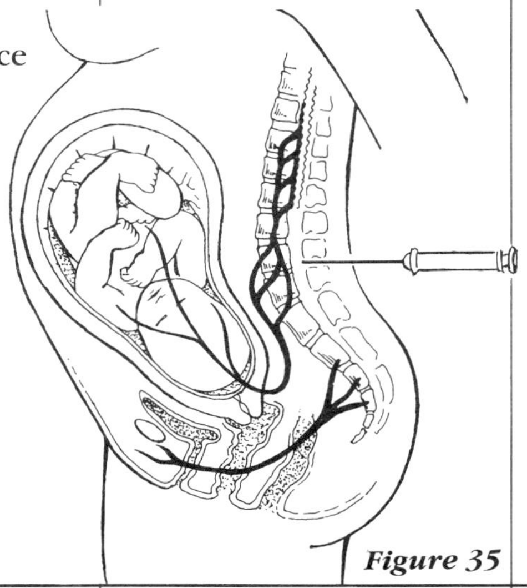

7 Choices and Variations in Labor and Birth

In this chapter, you will learn about—

- Informed consent.
- Medical procedures used in late pregnancy, labor, and birth.
- Variations and complications in labor.
- Cesarean birth.
- Vaginal birth after a cesarean birth.
- Coping with an unexpected outcome.

Every labor is different, as women who have had more than one child will tell you. Some labors are more challenging than others and can require more coaching and more attention to the techniques you have learned. Some labors require more medical intervention than others because of risks to the mother or the baby. Knowing what to expect in different situations will help you cope with whatever kind of labor you have. It is important to stay flexible and to have confidence in yourself and in those you have chosen to help you give birth. If you don't understand something, ask, and get the information you need.

Informed Consent

It is your right as a patient to be informed about any medical care you receive during labor and delivery and after the baby is born. This means that your health care provider must—

◆ Explain any procedure being done.
◆ Tell you why it is being done.
◆ Tell you what choices you have.
◆ Inform you about the risks of any procedure.
◆ Consider your preferences.

It is better to discuss common procedures your health care provider will use for labor and birth before you go into labor, perhaps at 30 to 34 weeks. Obviously this is not possible for some emergency procedures. Ask as many questions as you can. Let your health care provider know what is important to you. Ask your provider to write your requests about your care on your medical record. You also can bring your written requests in and have your provider keep them as part of your record. Be sure to keep a copy for yourself.

Medical Procedures in Late Pregnancy, Labor, and Birth

Some common medical procedures done during late pregnancy, labor, and birth are discussed below.

Late Pregnancy

During late pregnancy, any of the following tests may be done to check the condition of the baby. These are not done for all pregnancies.

◆ **Ultrasound**—An ultrasound exam uses sound waves to make a two-dimensional picture of the baby on a screen. (The picture is called a sonogram.) The picture may be used to determine the number of babies, the location of the placenta, and the position or the age (how many weeks) of the baby. It can be done at any point in your pregnancy. Though no side effects of ultrasound are evident, the long-term effects to the baby are unknown.

◆ **Nonstress test**—This test uses an electronic fetal monitor to check the well-being of the baby. It may be done when the baby is overdue or if there is any concern about the health of the baby or the mother. The test measures how the baby responds to his or her own body movements. Normally, the heart rate of a baby increases as he or she moves, just as your heart rate increases when you are more active. If the baby's heart rate increases as he or she moves, the test is called "reactive"; if it does not increase, the test is called "nonreactive."

A nonstress test can be done in a doctor's office, clinic, or hospital. During a nonstress test, the pregnant woman has two belts placed around her abdomen—one to monitor the baby's heart rate and one to measure any activity of the uterus. Whenever the baby moves, the woman presses a button that marks the movement on the paper recording of the fetal heart rate. Usually, the nonstress test takes 20 to 30 minutes. It is painless.

◆ **Contraction stress test**—This test measures the response of the baby's heart rate when the uterus contracts. It is usually done if the nonstress test is nonreactive. Mild contractions of the uterus are induced by using a drug called oxytocin or by having the mother stimulate her nipples. The baby's heart rate in response to the contractions is then recorded. The test is normal (negative) if the baby's heart rate responds as if the mother were in labor.

Risks of the test include the premature onset of labor (very rare) or unnecessary intervention if the results indicate a problem when none exists. The contraction stress test is invasive if it involves introducing medication into the body. Risks of not doing the test are that problems with the baby might not be discovered.

◆ **Biophysical profile**—This test uses a nonstress test and an ultrasound test to measure five components of fetal health: the fetal heart rate, fetal movement, fetal muscle tone, fetal breathing movements, and the amount of amniotic fluid. Each of these is given a score of zero to two, so the highest possible score is 10. This test is done when

there are concerns about the health of the baby in the last few weeks before birth. It is noninvasive and is usually done in a medical office or clinic.

Labor

Following are some procedures that are often used during labor. You should discuss with your health care provider which of these he or she commonly uses, the reasons for their use, and your own preferences.

◆ **Electronic fetal monitor**—This monitor is used to check the response of the baby to labor. Information about the baby's heart rate and the uterine contractions is recorded on a long strip of paper. It indicates how the baby's heart rate reacts to contractions.

An **external fetal monitor** consists of a small instrument that measures the baby's heart rate and a small instrument that measures the contractions of the uterus. The two instruments are held in place with belts around the woman's abdomen. It is difficult for a woman to move around freely with the external monitor because each time she moves, the belts have to be adjusted *(Fig. 36)*.

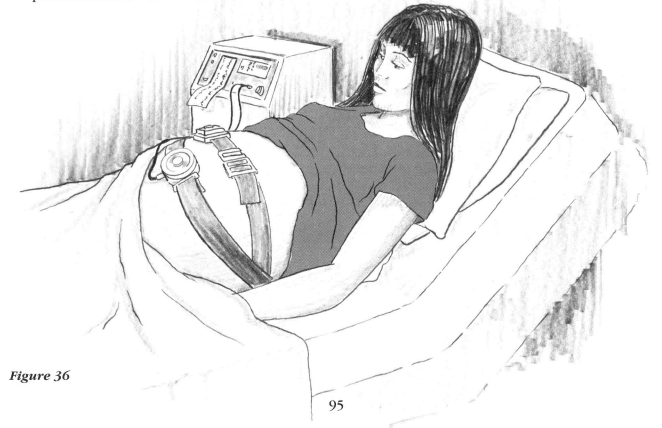

Figure 36

An **internal fetal monitor** consists of an electrode that is attached to the baby's scalp to measure the baby's heart rate. It may also include a thin tube (called a catheter) that is inserted through the vagina into the uterus to measure the strength of uterine contractions. This internal catheter is more accurate than the external instrument. Internal monitoring can be done only after the cervix has begun to dilate and after the membranes (bag of waters) are broken. A woman with an internal monitor is usually confined to bed, but she has more freedom of movement than a woman with an external monitor *(Fig. 37)*.

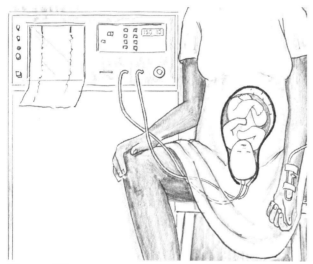

Figure 37

Sometimes a combination of electronic fetal monitoring methods is used. For example, an internal scalp electrode may be used to measure the fetal heart rate and an external belt used to monitor contractions of the uterus. Many health care providers use constant electronic fetal monitoring for every patient. Others may monitor women who are having a normal labor for only 20 minutes an hour. Women with high-risk labors will be monitored constantly, either by a special stethoscope or electronically.

Current research does not support the need for constant electronic monitoring throughout labor for all low-risk pregnancies.

You may wish to ask your health care provider if you can be monitored only now and then throughout labor, so that you have more freedom of movement. Ask your health care provider about his or her preferences for monitoring and the reasons for them.

◆ **Perineal shave ("prep")**—Some health care providers believe that during labor pubic hair around a woman's perineum should be clipped or shaved to prevent infection. Many health care providers believe that this is unnecessary and may even increase the chance of infection. Routine prep is becoming rare in current practice.

◆ **Enema**—A small enema may be given in early labor to prevent contamination or to stimulate labor. This is not necessary for all women in labor and is not usually ordered routinely.

◆ **IV (intravenous)**—A needle connected to a bag of fluids that is put into a vein in the woman's hand or arm is called an IV. An IV is used to prevent a woman in labor from becoming dehydrated (many women are not allowed fluids during labor) and to provide some energy for working with the labor. It can also be used to administer drugs swiftly, directly into the bloodstream, if they are needed. The IV can be put on a portable pole so that the woman can walk with it. It limits mobility somewhat, and the insertion may be uncomfortable. Many health care providers use IVs only if the woman is dehydrated, is high risk, or is having a cesarean birth.

◆ **Amniotomy**—Breaking the bag of waters by the health care provider is called an amniotomy. This may be done to start labor or, in active labor, to speed the labor. It may also be done to insert an internal fetal monitor or to assess the color of amniotic fluid. It is painless. The health care provider uses a plastic instrument called an amniohook, which looks like a knitting needle, to break the membranes *(Fig. 38)*. When the membranes break, the woman feels a gush of fluid and her contractions may get stronger and/or closer together.

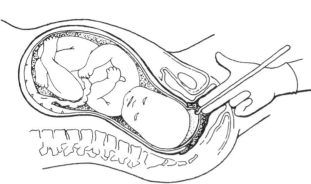

Figure 38

◆ **Induction of labor**—This means starting labor artificially. Labor may be induced because the bag of waters has broken but no contractions have come for several hours, because the baby is overdue, or because the mother has a medical condition (such as diabetes, pregnancy-induced hypertension, or heart disease) that makes an earlier delivery necessary.

For induction, a laboring woman will be given a medication called oxytocin (Pitocin) through her IV *(Fig. 39)*. If the cervix is not soft, a hormonal preparation (prostaglandin gel) may be put into the vagina to soften the cervix, which assists the progress of the labor. Electronic fetal monitoring is necessary during induction to detect contractions that are too close together or too strong. Contractions may be more intense than in noninduced labor and may require more advanced breathing and coping techniques and pain medication.

Oxytocin may also be given to increase the efficiency of contractions when labor is not progressing. This is called augmentation of labor.

Birth

Certain procedures may be done by the health care provider to help the baby during birth. These include—

◆ **Episiotomy**—This is an incision (cut) made right before birth at the bottom of the vagina toward the anus. It may be done directly toward or off to one side of the rectum *(Fig. 40)*. An episiotomy enlarges the opening of the vagina to prevent it from

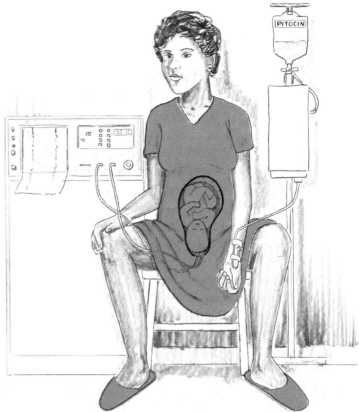

Figure 39

tearing when the baby is being born. An injection (local anesthesia) may be given where the incision is made so that the woman does not feel the incision or the repair. An episiotomy is not necessary for all births. It is more common with first births. After the birth, the episiotomy is sewn up with thread that dissolves so that the stitches do not have to be taken out.

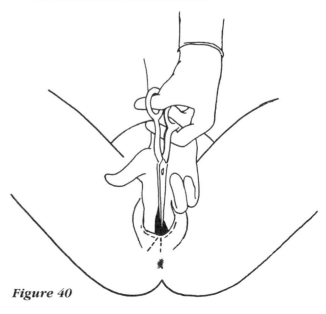

Figure 40

97

Many women and health care providers want to avoid an episiotomy if possible. Let your health care provider know if this is important to you. The application of warm, moist cloths and massage of the perineum during the latter part of pregnancy and during birth may help to avoid an episiotomy. Also, a side-lying position during delivery may put less strain on the tissues and help avoid an episiotomy.

◆ **Forceps**—Forceps are instruments that assist delivery of the baby's head *(Fig. 41)*. They may be used when the mother is too tired to push, when she has no urge to push because of the use of an epidural or caudal block, when the baby is in distress and has to be born immediately, or when the head has to be turned into a better position for birth. Anesthesia (local or pudendal block) is usually used to numb the vaginal area before the forceps are used. An episiotomy is usually necessary. Forceps may cause temporary bruising on the sides of the baby's face. This will fade in a few days.

◆ **Vacuum extraction**—A vacuum extractor is a cup-shaped device that fits on the baby's head *(Fig. 42)*. Suction is created between the cup and the head to help move the baby through the vagina. It is used for the same reasons that forceps are used. Sometimes the soft skin of the baby's head will be temporarily swollen from a vacuum extraction.

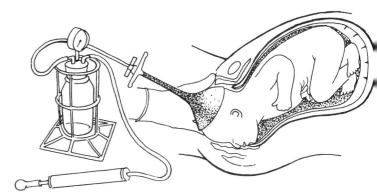

Figure 42

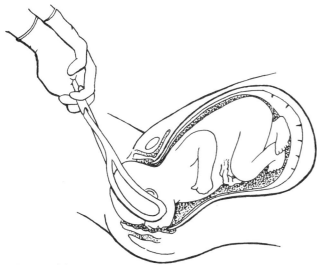

Figure 41

Variations and Complications in Labor

Whatever kind of labor you have, you and your labor companion should feel prepared to cope with it. This section discusses several variations on normal labor and special coping techniques you can use for each variation.

Short Labors

While they may seem ideal, short labors can be difficult. Often the contractions come on hard and strong from the beginning, making it more difficult to cope with them. If your labor is very short, you will need lots of support from your labor companion. You may have to use more rapid and shallow breathing rather than the slow breathing you would normally use in early labor. Make sure you breathe lightly to avoid hyperventilating. This goes for your labor companion too!

Women who have a short labor commonly feel cheated of the labor experience. Because it all went so fast, they might not remember much of the labor. If this happens to you, talk it over with your labor companion to help you put the pieces together.

down, it is difficult not to get discouraged. Here are some things you can do to help:

- ◆ Rest or sleep if possible (especially in prelabor and early labor).
- ◆ Practice a relaxation exercise.
- ◆ Walk to increase the strength of your contractions.
- ◆ Change your position frequently.
- ◆ Keep your bladder empty.
- ◆ Take showers or baths. (Take only showers if your bag of waters has broken.)
- ◆ Use visualization to picture the baby coming down and out, or your cervix opening up. Picture yourself working with your labor with renewed energy. (See page 80.)

Sometimes medical intervention is necessary in a long labor. The medication Pitocin may be necessary to stimulate labor. An IV may be necessary to provide fluid and prevent dehydration. More careful fetal monitoring is done to assess the condition of the baby. Pain medication is more likely to be given as the length of labor increases. If the baby is under stress, or if the labor has gone on for a very long time, the health care provider may decide that a cesarean birth is necessary.

When Baby Comes Fast

If you are not yet at the hospital and you feel that the baby is going to be born right away, don't race to get to the hospital. Stay calm, and call the emergency medical services system for help.

Some of the signs that the baby is going to be born right away are—

- ◆ A strong urge to bear down.
- ◆ Seeing the baby's head or any part of the baby's body at the vagina.
- ◆ Feeling the baby coming.

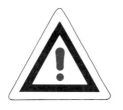

Long Labors

Long labors can occur in several forms. Some labors start slowly and proceed normally; some slow down in the middle; others may go along at a normal rate until the pushing phase, and then take a long time. Any time your labor slows

Back Labor (Posterior Position of the Baby)

Back labor usually occurs when the back of the baby's head is pressing against the mother's backbone. This is called a posterior presentation and may be more uncomfortable than normal labor. These labors may be slower because in this position the baby takes longer to progress through the pelvis and birth canal.

There are many ways to cope with back labor. Walking, pelvic rocking in a hands-and-knees position *(Fig. 43)*, side-lying *(Fig. 44)*, or sitting up and leaning forward *(Fig. 45a and b)* are all positions that may help you be more comfortable. If you have back labor, you should change positions frequently. Your position is very important because it can help move the baby off your back and help the baby turn into a better position for birth.

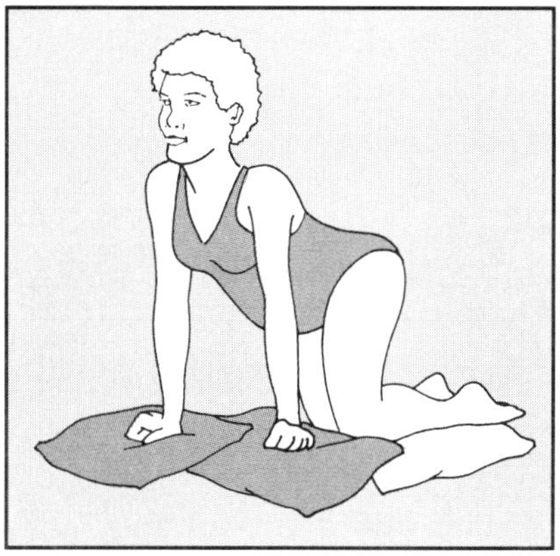

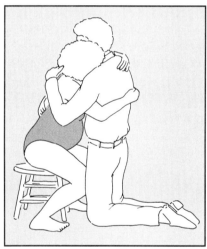

Figure 43

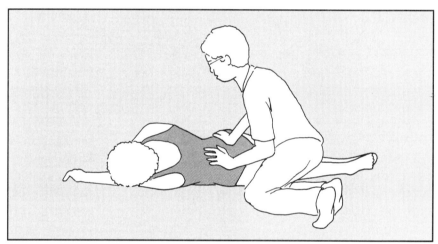

Figure 44

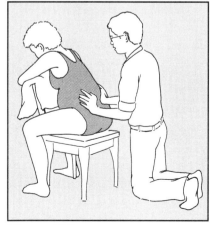

Figure 45a

Firm pressure against your lower back by your labor companion or a nurse is often helpful. This is called counterpressure and it is applied with the heel of the hand against the area where the woman feels the most discomfort. *(See Figures 44 and 45b.)*

Warm or cool packs against your lower back can also help. These are usually available in the labor and delivery area.

Figure 45b

100

Breech Presentation

About three percent of babies enter the birth canal with the buttocks or feet coming first. These babies are said to be breech. Breech babies may have problems during delivery. The umbilical cord may prolapse (slip through the cervix, possibly cutting off oxygen to the baby). The head may be delayed in being born because it is the largest part and hasn't had the opportunity to be molded by passing first through the pelvis and birth canal. The cord may get pinched between the baby's head and the mother's body. There are several choices to consider if your baby is breech, depending on your situation and the practice of your health care provider.

Your health care provider may teach you certain positions during pregnancy to encourage the baby to turn on his or her own. During late pregnancy, some health care providers may want to try to turn a breech baby around to a headfirst position. This is called external version. If your baby is breech, your health care provider will tell you if external version is a possibility for you. In this procedure, the baby is monitored and the mother is given medication to help relax the uterus so that the baby has room to turn. Then the health care provider presses on the abdomen to try to turn the baby to a headfirst position. Some babies turn easily, while others don't. This procedure is uncomfortable and requires that the health care provider be specially trained. Risks include fetal distress and, rarely, injury to the uterus.

In many cases, a cesarean is performed if a baby is breech. This is especially true if it is the woman's first baby, if her pelvis is small, or if the baby is large.

Cesarean Birth

Cesarean birth is the birth of a baby through a cut (incision) made in the mother's abdomen and uterus. The decision to perform a cesarean may be made before labor begins or at any time during labor if problems develop. The reasons a cesarean is performed include—

◆ The baby is too large to fit through the mother's pelvis.
◆ The baby is in distress.
◆ The baby is not in a good position for birth (breech or transverse position).
◆ The umbilical cord prolapses (drops into the vagina before the baby and cuts off the baby's oxygen supply). This is an emergency situation.
◆ There are problems with the placenta, for example, the placenta fully or partially covers the cervix (placenta previa) or the placenta separates from the wall of the uterus before the baby is born (abruptio placenta).
◆ The mother has an underlying condition, such as heart disease, pre-eclampsia, or diabetes. Active genital herpes at the time of labor is also a reason for a cesarean.
◆ The mother has had a cesarean before. This is not usually in itself an indication for another cesarean. (See "Vaginal Birth After Cesarean" on page 102.)

After the decision has been made to perform a cesarean, the woman's abdomen is cleaned with an antiseptic solution. Some of her pubic hair is shaved. A catheter is inserted into the bladder through the urethra to keep it empty during surgery. Anesthesia is given. This may be an epidural block, a spinal block, or general anesthesia. (See the chart that begins on page 89.) Many hospitals allow the labor companion to be present during surgery. If you have a cesarean, be sure to ask.

Generally, the baby is born 10 to 15 minutes after the cesarean operation has begun. It takes about 30 to 45 minutes to repair the incision. Incisions are made both in the abdominal area and into the uterus. Most incisions now are made horizontally—on the abdomen near the line of the pubic hair (called a bikini cut) and

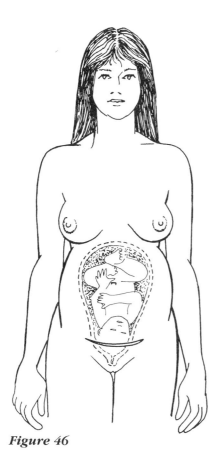

Figure 46

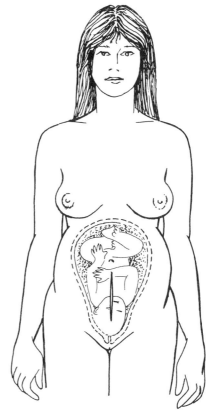

Figure 47

low on the uterus *(Fig. 46)*. However, vertical incisions *(Fig. 47)* are sometimes necessary because of the baby's position or the need for a quick delivery.

Recovery after a cesarean is slower than after a vaginal birth and usually requires a hospital stay of four to six days. When a woman who has had a cesarean gets home, she will need help with household chores for at least a month. Some women say that it takes a good six months for complete recovery following a cesarean. Eating well and getting plenty of rest will help speed recovery.

Vaginal Birth After Cesarean (VBAC)

The old saying "once a cesarean, always a cesarean" is currently being challenged. Many women who have a baby by cesarean can safely deliver subsequent babies vaginally if the following conditions are met:

◆ The reasons for the cesarean are not present in the subsequent pregnancy.
◆ The cesarean was done with a horizontal incision in the uterus.
◆ The mother and baby are closely monitored and the hospital is equipped to cope with high-risk situations.

Coping With the Unexpected

All parents worry at some point in the pregnancy that something will go wrong with their labor or with their baby. Usually these fears are groundless, but couples who have had unexpected outcomes often wish they had had more information about how to cope. Unexpected outcomes in labor can include feeling disappointed by your responses to labor, having a premature baby, having an unplanned cesarean birth, having a baby with birth defects or one in intensive care, or experiencing an infant's death.

In dealing with an unexpected outcome, parents should know that—

◆ It's normal to have mixed emotions.

◆ It's important to allow themselves to experience whatever feelings they have; none of their feelings is "bad."

◆ One day they will feel better, but they should give themselves time.

◆ Grief is experienced by each person in the family, so individual family members might not be available to each other for support. They may need outside help.

◆ Talking with other parents who have had similar experiences is helpful. (See "Helpful Organizations," Appendix F, for a list of self-help groups.)

◆ It's important for them to continue healthy eating habits, exercise, and whatever makes them feel good. Someone who is mentally and physically strong will be more able to cope than someone who is in poor health.

The Next Step

Now that you have completed Module II, you should start to get ready for your labor and birth. You should—

◆ Look over the "Choices in Childbirth" checklist (Appendix A) and begin to make decisions about your options. Discuss these with your health care provider and make a copy to take with you to the hospital.

◆ Take a tour of the labor/delivery area where you will have your baby.

◆ Practice your chosen coping skills for labor daily.

◆ Continue to eat well and to exercise.

◆ Look over the checklist on page 77 and do as many of these things as you can.

◆ Pack your labor bag.

Module III
Family and Infant Care

Who will the baby look like? Will we have a girl or a boy? What are we going to name this baby? These are all questions you are probably asking by now. In addition to these questions, as the parents of a newborn, you will continue to have many more about the baby's care, whether it is your first baby or one of many. And you will also be coping with the hormonal and physical changes that women experience after having a baby, as well as the emotional effects on the whole family. This module covers how to take care of your baby, yourself, and your family in the often-confusing postpartum period.

Chapter 8 discusses what to expect in the first few days after birth. It also includes information on breastfeeding and bottle feeding. Chapter 9 covers newborn care and the adjustments a family must make when a new baby arrives. Chapter 10 is about ensuring the health and safety of your baby. Chapter 11 discusses going back to work and family planning.

8 *After Your Baby Is Born*

In this chapter, you will learn
about—
◆ How your baby will look
   and act after birth.
◆ The physical and emotional
   changes that you may
   experience after the baby is
   born.
◆ Your postpartum care.
◆ Breastfeeding and bottle
   feeding your baby, and how
   to burp your baby.

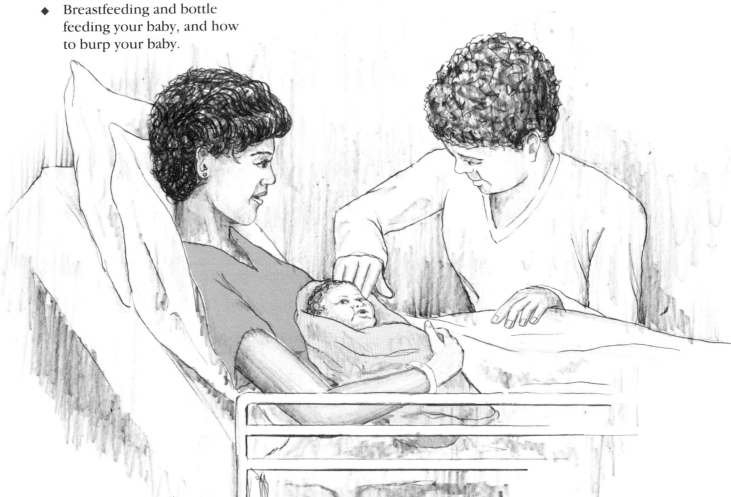

All parents remember the first time they saw their newborn baby. After so many months of waiting and dreaming, the baby is finally here. Often the excitement and joy overwhelms them; sometimes they are just exhausted and relieved that labor is over. Whatever their reactions may be, this is a day they will never forget.

This chapter covers the first six weeks after your baby is born—the postpartum period. It describes what to expect right after the delivery. It also describes how your baby will look and act and the physical and emotional changes you will experience. In addition, the chapter discusses some of the choices you will have about your baby's care in the hospital and about breastfeeding and bottle feeding. (See "Choices in Childbirth," Appendix A.) By thinking about these issues in advance, you will be able to make the decisions that are right for you.

Immediately After Birth

As soon as your baby is born, your health care provider will check the baby's basic condition and assign the baby an Apgar score. This score describes the baby's breathing, skin color, reflexes, heart rate, and activity.

Ideally, you will be given the baby to hold immediately after birth so you can begin forming an emotional bond right from the start. This is also the best time to start breastfeeding. Tell your health care provider in advance that you will want your baby with you right after birth, unless your baby's condition requires immediate care in the nursery.

If you had an episiotomy, it will be stitched up at this time. If you had a cesarean birth, the incision will be sutured. This takes 30 to 45 minutes. You may feel a little shaky or cold after you give birth; this is normal. If you do, ask the nurse for a warm blanket.

Caring for Your Baby in the Hospital

You may be able to have your baby "room in" with you while you are in the hospital. This means the baby stays in your room all day and all night, except for visiting hours. Some mothers prefer this because they can practice taking care of the baby and they know the baby is being fed and cuddled. Other mothers prefer to send their babies back to the nursery at night.

Some hospitals offer mother/baby nursing in which one nurse cares for the mother and baby together. The baby remains at the mother's bedside, and the nurse serves as a care giver, role model, and teacher.

If you are breastfeeding, you should feed the baby on demand both day and night to encourage milk production. The nurse may ask if you want the baby to be given bottles of formula between breastfeedings. This is not a good idea since it means your baby will nurse less often and not be as hungry for breastmilk. Therefore, your milk supply will not build up. Also, a baby uses different sucking techniques to get milk from a bottle and from the breast. A baby who is given a bottle before his or her nursing habits are well established may reject the breast in favor of the bottle. Wait until the baby is four to six weeks old before introducing a bottle for any feedings, or discuss this with the baby's health care provider.

Hello, Baby!

Your baby's appearance at birth may surprise you! The head may be elongated or molded from the pressures of birthing *(Fig. 48)*. Don't worry; it will return to a normal shape within a week.

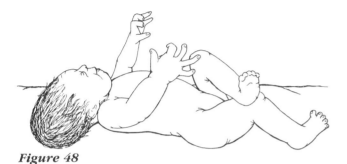

Figure 48

You will also notice the fontanels, or "soft spots," on the baby's head—areas where the bones of the skull have not joined together *(Fig. 49)*. These are covered by a very tough membrane, and there is no danger of hurting them when you touch the baby's head or wash the baby's hair.

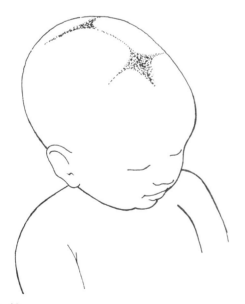

Figure 49

The baby's skin will be wrinkled and loose and may be flaky. The skin may be covered with a fine layer of downy hair, called lanugo, and with a white, cheesy-looking substance called vernix, which protected the baby's skin in the womb. It also is normal for the hands and feet to be bluish for a time until the blood flow is well established.

The baby's eyes may be red and puffy from the pressures of birth, and the eye drops put in after birth may also irritate the eyes. In both sexes the baby's genitals and breasts may be swollen for several days after birth. This is due to hormones that pass from the mother's system to the baby's just before birth. The swollen breasts may contain some milk, and girl infants may have a slight, bloody discharge from their vagina. Neither condition is a cause for worry and both will go away when the swelling does.

The umbilical cord, which was clamped and cut at birth, will look like a dark tag of skin covering the belly button. It will drop off within about two weeks. For instructions on how to care for the cord, see page 130.

Other conditions your baby may have include—

◆ Birthmarks, which may also develop in the first month of life. Most will disappear or fade by the time the child is of school age.

◆ Mongolian spots, which are patches of dark-blue skin on a baby's body, often on the lower back. They occur most often in families of black, oriental, or Mediterranean origin. These spots are completely harmless and usually disappear by the time the child enters school.

◆ A small blister on the upper lip, caused by intense sucking on hands or fingers in the womb.

◆ A hematoma (swelling caused by blood and other fluid beneath the scalp), which will usually disappear in about a week.

◆ Small, white spots on the baby's nose, chin, and cheeks (milia). These are caused by undeveloped or blocked sweat glands. They disappear over time. Your baby may also have other rashes, splotches, or pimples on the chest, back, or face which will go away on their own. Don't put any medications on these spots—they will only irritate the baby's skin.

Your baby may have newborn jaundice soon after he or she is born. Jaundice, which may cause your baby's skin to have a yellow tint, occurs when red blood cells break down and the by-products of this breakdown are carried through the bloodstream. Bilirubin is the name of these by-products. If the jaundice does not disappear on its own, the baby may be put under special lights that help to break down the bilirubin. Your baby's level of bilirubin may be monitored with blood tests after birth, but only rarely is newborn jaundice a cause for real concern. Premature or ill babies are more at risk for physiologic jaundice. There are also other rarer causes of jaundice.

If you have a baby boy, you may have the option of having him circumcised before you leave the hospital. Circumcision is usually done the day after the baby is born, provided he weighs enough and is healthy. Medical opinion is divided on whether circumcision is beneficial or not. You can get more information on circumcision from your health care provider or the class instructor.

The Sensational Newborn

Even though newborns are unable to talk, they are very aware of the world around them. Their senses of touch, sight, hearing, taste, and smell are active from the day they are born. You may be surprised to see how responsive your baby is to you in the first weeks after birth. You will soon discover that your baby has personal preferences for how he or she is held, played with, and fed.

A newborn's sense of touch is very sensitive. Newborns like to be held softly but firmly, and they like to be warm. Holding them closely, wrapped in a blanket, or rocking them will often calm them when they are fussy.

A newborn sees most clearly at a distance of 8 to 12 inches, or just about the distance between your face and the baby's when you are cuddling or feeding him or her. Babies like to look at human faces. They are also attracted to black-and-white contrasts.

A newborn's hearing is very well developed. Babies especially like high-pitched voices and sounds that are soft and rhythmic, like a lullaby.

Newborns prefer sweet tastes and have a very good sense of smell. They have been shown to recognize the scent of their mother's breastmilk from among other mothers' on identical cloths.

Babies are born with certain behaviors and reactions that are meant to help them survive outside the womb. Some of them are—

◆ The startle (Moro) reflex—Babies surprised by sudden changes in light, noise, movement, or position will fling out their arms and legs, then quickly pull them back onto their chest while curling their body as if to cling. This is their way of saying there is too much light, noise, or movement and of reminding you to be gentler.

◆ The rooting reflex—If you stroke a baby's cheek or lips, the baby's head will turn in the direction of the stroking and his or her mouth will search for a nipple. This helps the baby receive nourishment.

◆ The sucking reflex—If you touch a baby's mouth or cheek with your finger or nipple, the baby will pucker his or her lips and try to suck it. This is how a baby is able to latch on to a nipple and feed.

Babies have six basic states of awareness or consciousness. They are—

◆ Heavy sleep—In the first weeks of life, babies sleep on and off all day long. A baby sleeping heavily will not be awakened easily, even at the sound of normal household noises. In fact, it is a good idea to let your baby nap in a safe place near the center of family activity so that the baby gets used to sleeping with some noise around.

◆ Light sleep—A baby who is sleeping lightly may move and make noises and may have slightly opened eyes.

◆ Drowsy—A drowsy baby is not yet asleep and may respond to your presence or to noise. The baby may wake up and then return to sleep. Although you may enjoy having your baby take "cat naps" on your lap throughout the day, your life will be easier to organize if the baby learns the difference between sleep and awake time. When the baby is drowsy, put him or her in the crib or carriage to nap. When the baby is awake, take him or her out of the crib.

- Quiet alert—Babies have two awake states, quiet alert and active alert. In the quiet alert state, your baby will be wide-eyed and able to focus on your face or a toy. This is the best time to play with your baby.
- Active alert—In the active alert state, your baby will move around more and may be fussy. A baby in this state will usually be happier if playtime stops and he or she is comforted to a less active state.
- Crying—Babies spend a lot of time crying in the early weeks and months. This is a way of talking to you. A crying baby should not be left to "cry it out," but should be picked up and taken care of right away. Crying may mean that a diaper needs to be changed or that the baby is hungry, bored, or in need of a change of position.

You cannot spoil a baby! The baby will learn to trust you if you respond quickly every time he or she cries. Babies whose needs are met quickly in the first few months are less likely to be fussy and irritable later on. Your baby needs to be held, cuddled, walked, rocked, and talked to softly. Front-pack carriers are an easy way to give your baby physical contact while leaving your hands free.

Postpartum Changes in the Mother

Your body changes rapidly after delivery. Your uterus will return to its normal state in six weeks, but it might take longer for the rest of you to feel "back to normal" again.

In the first few postpartum days you will lose, through urination and perspiration, much of the extra fluid gained during pregnancy. Try to empty your bladder every two hours, even if you don't feel a strong urge to do so.

If you are breastfeeding, you might notice that you have contractions when you nurse your baby. These are called "after-pains." They occur because hormones are released during nursing that help the uterus shrink. You will have a vaginal discharge for several weeks. It begins as

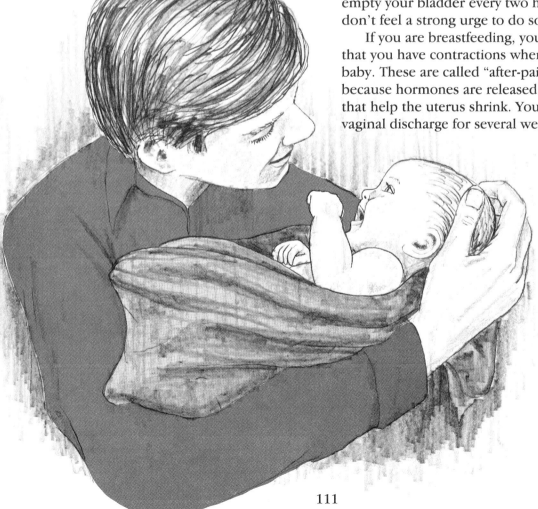

bright red, fades to brownish and pinkish, and then becomes white over time. If you begin to bleed heavily—such that you soak two sanitary pads in one hour—or if you pass blood clots, call your health care provider.

Menstruation will return in six to eight weeks after delivery if you do not breastfeed. For women who do breastfeed, the time when menstruation returns varies greatly. Remember, even if you do not menstruate, you may be ovulating, so do not rely on breastfeeding as a method of family planning. For more information on postpartum family planning, see Chapter 11.

If you had an episiotomy, it may cause you discomfort for a week or two. Follow your health care provider's instructions for relieving the discomfort. If it doesn't get better within two weeks, or if you notice any swelling or redness, or if you have a fever, call your health care provider.

Whether or not you are breastfeeding, your breasts will feel heavier than normal due to the engorgement that occurs when your milk comes in. You may find you need a bra with good support both day and night to be comfortable. If you are not breastfeeding, you can use ice packs on your breasts or take a mild pain reliever to reduce the discomfort. The engorgement will go away in a week or two. If you are breastfeeding, the discomfort can be relieved by nursing your baby very often during the first weeks. For more information on breastfeeding, see pages 114–120.

Emotionally, the days after birth may seem like a roller coaster. You may be full of energy and excitement one minute, and depressed or crying the next. This has much to do with the physical and hormonal changes your body is going through, as well as the stress of taking care of a new baby and the lack of sleep. Accept your emotions and don't take them too seriously. Ask your partner, friends, and relatives for support when you need it.

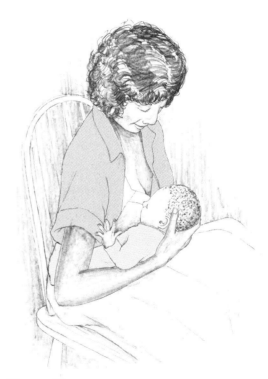

Figure 50

For Fathers

You are also physically and emotionally affected by the birth of your baby. You may feel tired due to loss of sleep, overwhelmed by new responsibilities, left out as the attention shifts to the baby, or just very excited. Try to accept the emotional turmoil as normal. Don't expect to have it all together right away. Becoming a father for the first time or adding another child to your family changes your life tremendously. It will take some time before you adjust to the changes.

Common Postpartum Discomforts

Listed below are some of the common discomforts that women feel after childbirth and things you can do to feel better.

Discomfort	What You Should Do	Danger Signs*
Abdominal cramping, after-pains, especially while nursing	Practice relaxation breathing or ask your health care provider for medication if pains are severe.	None.
Vaginal bleeding	Wear sanitary pads (no tampons).	Heavy bleeding, passing clots.
Episiotomy stitches	Pour warm water over stitches each time you use the bathroom, or apply ice packs during first 24 hours. After that time, try sitting in a bathtub with warm water. Avoid sitting in soapy water, as it may irritate the incision.	Any swelling, redness, or fever. Severe pain in the perineal area.
Constipation	Eat high-fiber foods and drink plenty of water or fruit juice, especially prune juice.	Inability to have a bowel movement.
Hemorrhoids	Apply witch hazel compresses, do Kegel exercises, sit on firm surfaces.	None.
Abdominal soreness after cesarean birth	Hold a pillow or press down gently with your hands on area of incision when moving, coughing, laughing, or nursing baby. Nursing mothers should also try the "football" hold (*Fig. 50*). While you are in the hospital, pain medication is available from medical staff.	Any redness, swelling, or fever.

* If you experience any of these danger signs or chills or abdominal pain, contact your health care provider immediately.

Exercise and Physical Activity

Women who have delivered vaginally should have no problem moving around soon after birth. You should be careful getting out of bed the first time. Call someone to help you since you may be a little dizzy. Do not begin, or resume, any exercise program more strenuous than walking until you have spoken with your health care provider.

If you had a cesarean delivery, remember that, in addition to recovering from childbirth, you have to recover from major abdominal surgery. The nursing staff will assist you the first couple of times you get out of bed after a cesarean birth. After that, you will be encouraged to walk frequently, but to take it slowly. You will need your strength to take care of the baby. After your health care provider gives you the go-ahead, you can begin an exercise program.

Feeding Your Baby

Feeding a baby means more than providing nutritional food. Your touch, the sound of your voice, and the affectionate look in your eye will give your baby emotional nourishment. Babies cannot thrive on food alone. They need your loving attention to grow and develop properly.

It is a good idea to decide which method of feeding you wish to use before your baby is born so that you can be prepared. The advantages of breastfeeding and of bottle feeding are discussed below. If you decide to breastfeed, you can always introduce a bottle for some of the feedings once your milk supply is well established, usually in four to six weeks. However, if you bottle feed first, it will be difficult or sometimes impossible to switch to breastfeeding.

Advantages of Breastfeeding
Medical professionals endorse breastmilk as the most nutritious food for a baby. In addition to receiving nutritional benefits, nursing babies enjoy a special closeness with their mother. Among other reasons, breastfeeding is advantageous because—

- Breast milk is more easily digested than formula and it has the right balance of nutrients for the baby.
- Breastfeeding helps the baby avoid allergies.
- Breastfeeding transfers the mother's antibodies and friendly bacteria to the baby to help keep the baby from getting sick.
- Breastfed babies tend to have fewer colds and milder illnesses.
- Breastfeeding is convenient.
- Breastfeeding is less expensive than bottle feeding.

Advantages of Bottle Feeding
There are several brands and types of infant formula available today, all of which provide good nutrition for babies. Some of the reasons bottle feeding can be advantageous are because—

- Bottle-fed babies can be fed by someone other than the mother, so that a father, another family member, or friend can take an active part in feeding the baby.
- If the mother is taking medication, the baby will not be affected.
- The mother can begin to diet if she wishes without affecting the baby.

Breastfeeding Facts and Tips

If you decide to breastfeed, here is some basic information on how breastfeeding works and a few tips on getting started.

A basic fact of breastfeeding is the more you nurse, the more milk you make. Newborn babies usually want to nurse every 1–1/2 to 3 hours for the first two weeks or so.

Most of the difficulties in breastfeeding occur in the first few weeks, when you are unsure of yourself and learning something new. Breastfeeding is a natural thing to do, but it is also a learned skill for the woman and the baby. Having support will help you feel better and enjoy the experience more. It is worth it to "hang in there" and keep trying if you are having difficulties. The rewards and satisfaction of being this close to your baby more than make up for any initial problems you may have.

114

Some women have nipples that are inverted, either flat or folded in. Women with inverted nipples have problems nursing since it is difficult for a baby to latch on to an inverted nipple. To find out if your nipples are inverted, hold your breast at the edge of the areola between your thumb and forefinger and press in gently while pulling your fingers away from each other. If the nipple seems to disappear within the breast, it is inverted. Your health care provider can show you some simple exercises to correct this condition.

Anatomy and Physiology of the Breast

The breast is composed of glands, called alveoli, where the milk is produced. The milk made in these glands moves down and is stored in areas called milk sinuses, which are located behind the areola (the brown area surrounding the nipple) *(Fig. 51)*. When the baby sucks on the areola, a message is sent to the mother's brain and hormones are released which cause the milk to flow out of the nipple. This is called the let-down reflex.

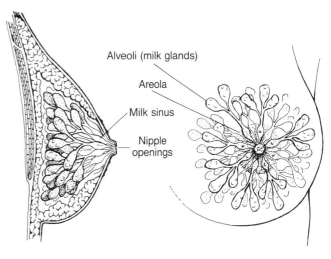

Figure 51

Getting Started

Get yourself in a comfortable, relaxed position. *Figures 52, 53, 54, and 55* show some of the positions for breastfeeding.

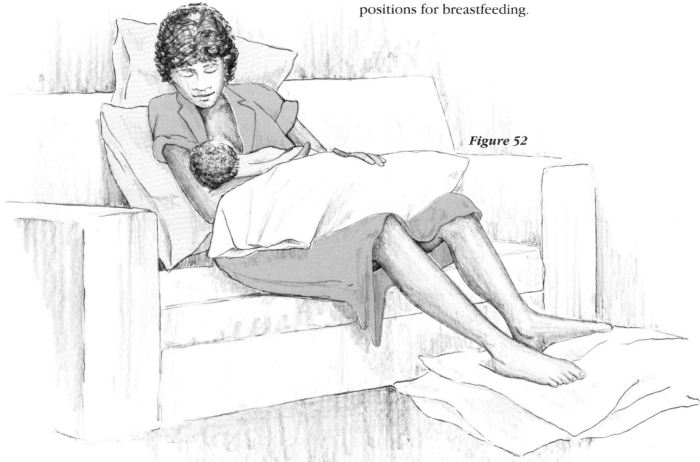

Figure 52

Hold your baby so that the baby's chest faces your breast and the tip of the baby's nose and chin touch your breast. Bring the baby up to your breast rather than bending over to the baby.

To get the baby onto the breast, tickle the baby's cheek with your nipple. The baby's head will then turn toward the breast (the rooting reflex).

When the baby opens his or her mouth wide, put the entire nipple in it. Be sure to get most of the dark part surrounding the nipple (the areola) into the baby's mouth. The milk pools which store the milk are located behind the areola and must have pressure put on them to get the milk flowing. Also, your nipples will get very sore if only the nipple is in the baby's mouth.

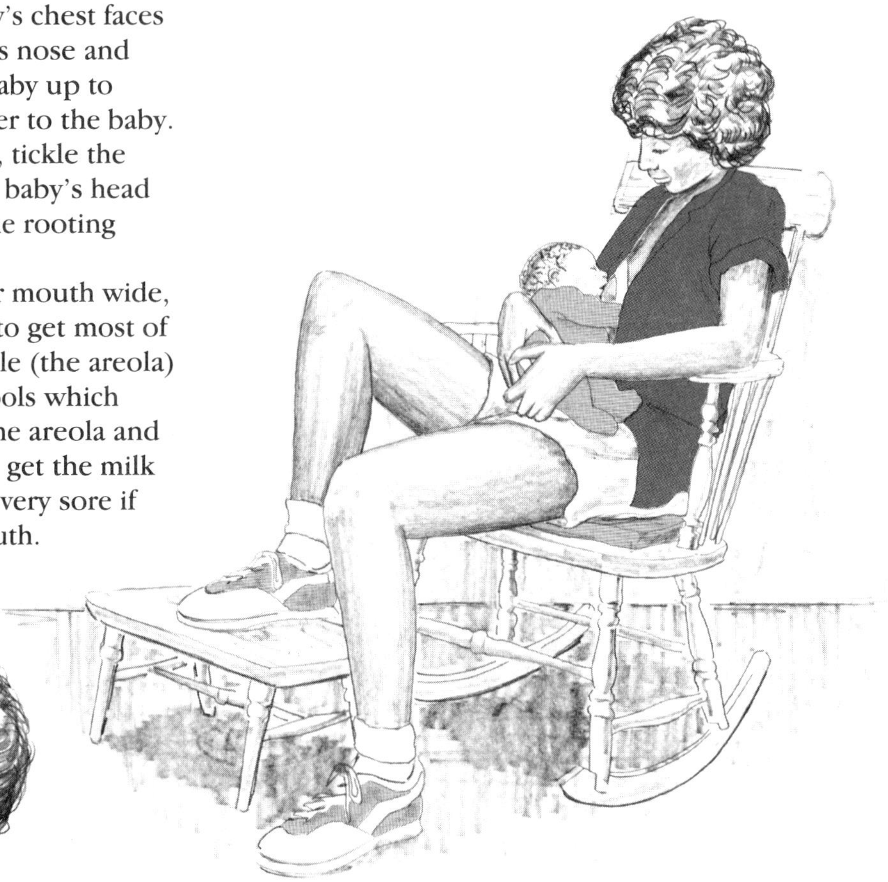

Figure 53

As the baby sucks on the nipple, your let-down reflex will begin. This may feel like a tingling sensation in your chest. It usually stops after the baby nurses for a few minutes.

You may want to begin nursing your baby for 5 minutes at each breast on the first day, 10 minutes on the second day, and 15 minutes or longer (depending on how long the baby wants to nurse) on the third day and thereafter. Babies nurse in bursts, not continuously. Long pauses in the baby's sucking pattern are normal. When the baby's sucking pattern slows, switch breasts.

To take your baby off the breast, put one finger into the corner of the baby's mouth and between the gums to break the suction and gently pull out your nipple.

Be sure the baby nurses from both breasts so that milk production is stimulated equally. It is a good idea to begin nursing on the breast taken

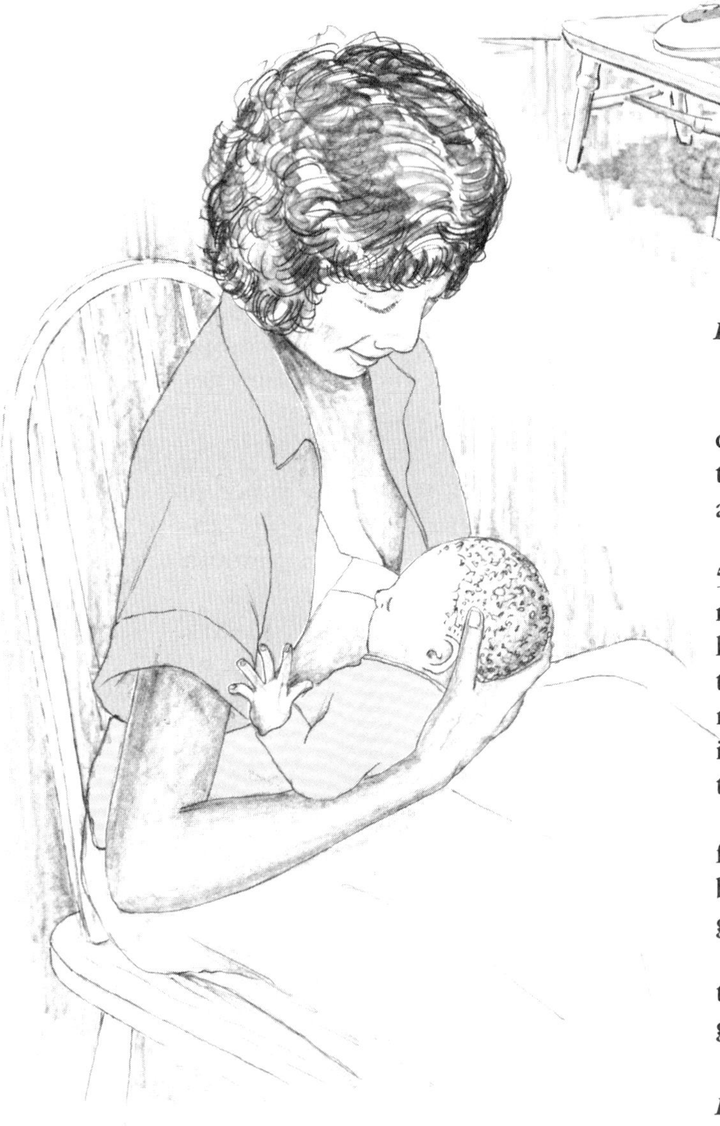

Figure 54

116

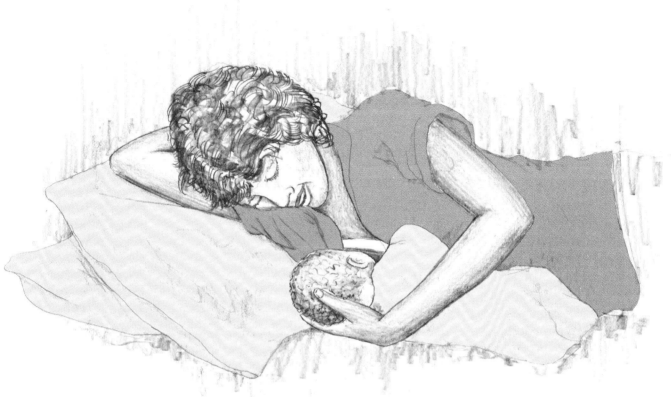

Figure 55

last on the previous feeding to ensure equal stimulation. You can put a safety pin on your bra to mark the breast nursed last so you know that is the one to start on next time.

Breastfeeding and Diet

You will need another 200 calories over your pregnancy diet to maintain your milk supply, and six to eight glasses of water, milk, or juice daily. An eight-ounce carton of yogurt contains 200 calories, so it isn't that much more than you were eating before. The most important thing is to continue eating a healthy diet and drinking plenty of fluids. This is not the time to diet.

You should avoid drinking alcoholic beverages or excess amounts of caffeinated beverages while you are breastfeeding. Talk to your health care provider before taking **any** over-the-counter or prescription drugs. Many are safe to be taken while breastfeeding, but you should check before taking anything.

Preventing and Treating Possible Problems

With some preparation and good support, most breastfeeding mothers have few problems. Mothers may have minor problems, which seem major at the time, that can be prevented or solved with simple solutions. The best and easiest way to treat problems in breastfeeding is to prevent the problems from happening. Below are suggestions for keeping your nipples healthy and for taking care of them if they get sore.

Keeping Nipples Healthy

To keep your nipples healthy—

◆ Be sure your baby is positioned properly for nursing, with the baby's body close to and facing yours and his or her mouth covering all or a good part of the areola.

◆ Change the baby's position each time you nurse so that the baby's mouth won't be touching the exact same place on your breast each time.

◆ Break the baby's suction at the breast with your finger. After feeding, express a little breastmilk and coat the nipple and areola with it. It has natural healing properties.

◆ After a feeding, air-dry your nipples for at least five minutes, or use a hair dryer on a low setting for 20 to 30 seconds. It is a good idea to let your nipples remain exposed to the air as often as possible to keep the skin dry and healthy.

◆ **Do not** wear rubber or soft plastic nipple

shields to protect your nipples from the baby's sucking. They rarely help the soreness, and they can keep your breasts from getting enough stimulation to produce milk.

◆ Don't use soap or other drying substances, such as alcohol, witch hazel, or tincture of benzoin, on your nipples.

Sore Nipples

If your nipples do get sore, act immediately to take care of them. You should—

◆ Nurse your baby more frequently, but for shorter periods of time.

◆ Limit sucking time to five minutes on the sore side, or on both sides if both are sore.

◆ Hand-express or pump a little milk so that your breasts don't get too full if your baby sleeps through a feeding.

◆ Offer the less-sore breast first most of the time, since the baby won't suck as hard when the second breast is offered.

◆ Take the baby off the affected breast for 24 to 48 hours, in the rare case that the soreness continues to worsen until the nipple cracks and bleeds and it is too painful to nurse. Nurse on the other breast, and express milk from the sore breast. Gradually resume nursing with five-minute sessions on the sore breast, starting twice a day. You can take acetaminophen or aspirin for pain about half an hour before a feeding.

Sometimes sore nipples are caused by thrush, a fungus infection in the baby's mouth. If you have sore nipples, look in the baby's mouth before nursing to see if there are milky white spots or a coating on the tongue, gums, or insides of the cheeks. Sometimes you cannot see any patches in the baby's mouth but there is enough of the fungus to give you very sore nipples. If the soreness persists between feedings, so that even a bra touching your nipple is very painful, call your health care provider. You will be given some medication for the baby's mouth, and the condition should clear up soon. You do not have to stop nursing.

Engorgement

Two to five days after childbirth you may experience swollen breasts caused by an increase of blood and fluid in the breast tissue and the incoming milk supply. This is called engorgement. The breasts may be hard, warm, and painful to the touch. The swelling makes it difficult for the baby to latch on to the nipple. The best way to prevent engorgement is to nurse frequently, on demand.

If you feel some engorgement in spite of frequent nursing, try putting warm compresses on your breasts or taking a warm bath or shower, and then hand-express some milk right before the baby nurses. This will make it easier for the baby to latch on to the nipple and will work out any lumps that might clog the ducts. See page 149 for directions on how to hand-express milk.

Engorgement goes away easily after the baby starts nursing well and frequently.

Clogged Duct

If you find a small lump on your breast that is warm, red, and painful to the touch, you may have a clogged milk duct. You should treat this right away to prevent a breast infection. To treat a clogged duct—

◆ Breastfeed more often and for a longer time on the affected side so that the breast is well emptied.

◆ Change your position for each feeding so that pressure is put on all parts of the breast and all ducts are emptied.

◆ Apply moist heat (warm, moist washcloths) to the affected breast several times a day.

◆ Do not put any pressure on the breast by sleeping on your stomach or by wearing tight bras or shirts.

If the lump does not go away in three days, see your health care provider.

Breast Infection

Symptoms of a breast infection (mastitis) include headache, a painful area or redness in the breast, a breast that is hot and tender to the touch, fever, and a general aching, flu-like feeling. A breast infection could be the result of a clogged duct or of another infection contracted by the mother.

If you think you have a breast infection, call your health care provider right away. You may be treated with antibiotics that are safe to take while you continue to nurse. It is not desirable or necessary to stop nursing when a breast is infected. In fact, stopping suddenly will worsen your condition. Comfort measures to use for a breast infection include—

◆ Resting as much as possible. Stay in bed with your baby and nurse every 2 to 2–1/2 hours.

◆ Applying moist heat to the breast. (Do not apply anything cold to an infected breast.)

◆ Taking acetaminophen or aspirin for discomfort and/or fever.

◆ Having the baby nurse at the affected breast first so that it can be emptied more completely.

◆ Wearing a firm, but not too tight, bra for support.

Breastfeeding and Sexuality

Breastfeeding makes some women feel more sexy. Other women may feel tired or "touched out" by nursing and caring for a baby all day long; they might not feel like being touched by their partner. Some men are turned on by the changes in a nursing woman's breasts; others may feel they are for the baby and "off limits" to him. Whatever your feelings are, be sure to talk about them with your partner. Good communication can help avoid misunderstandings and hurt feelings.

Breastfeeding Questions

How will I know if my baby is getting enough milk?

Even when a mother and baby are doing well with breastfeeding, some parents worry that their baby is not getting enough milk. It is difficult to judge how much milk a breastfed baby gets, since you do not see it. It is safe to say that a baby who wets six diapers a day, feeds 6 to 10 times a day, and sucks 10 minutes or more on each breast is getting enough to eat. Drinking liquids and nursing the baby more frequently builds up your milk supply.

I have small breasts. Will I be able to make enough milk for my baby?

The size of your breasts has nothing to do with how much milk you are able to produce.

Especially for Fathers

Breastfeeding is a wonderful gift of love to your new baby. The support, care, and love you give your partner will have much to do with how successful the experience is.

It is normal for fathers of breastfed babies to feel left out or even jealous of the closeness the mother and baby share when they are nursing. You can feel more involved by bringing the baby to the mother for feeding, by getting her something to drink while she's nursing, and by holding the baby after feedings and burping the baby if needed. You can also do more of the household chores and shopping to let her have some rest. She will need lots of help to get off to a good start breastfeeding. And once her milk supply is well established, you can, if you want to, give the baby a bottle with breastmilk or formula for some of the feedings.

Talk about your feelings with your partner so that resentment and bad feelings don't have a chance to grow. It is important to remember that you do not have to feed the baby to have a close relationship. The time you spend bathing, playing with, or massaging your baby will be very special to both of you. You can find ways to take care of your baby that will make you realize that the father's role in a baby's life is just as important and rewarding as the mother's.

Where can I get more information on or help with breastfeeding?

Hospitals and clinics often have consultants or nurses who can assist you with breastfeeding concerns. There are several good books about breastfeeding (see Appendix G) and a support and information group for breastfeeding mothers called the La Leche League. The La Leche League has local groups all across the country and around the world, and many offer telephone support. For women unable to locate a La Leche League in their area, finding other breastfeeding mothers to talk with is very important.

How can I keep breastfeeding when I return to work?

Many working mothers continue to breastfeed and to enjoy the special warmth and closeness with their baby. Breastfeeding for a working mother requires some planning. More information on breastfeeding after you return to work is in Chapter 11.

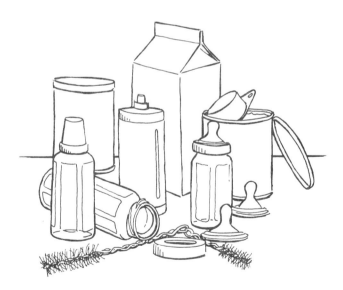

If you decide to bottle feed, here is some basic information on what you should know and what you will need.

Formula

Several types of infant formula are available today. Most formulas use nonfat cow's milk as their base; others use soy protein. Soy-based formulas are for babies with a milk allergy or intolerance. Some health care providers prefer using soy formulas for all babies.

Although there are few differences between the various milk-based formulas, some babies do better on one than on another. If your baby has gas, vomiting (not just spitting up), or bowel movement problems with one formula, ask your health provider to recommend another type.

Formula is available in several forms. Ready-to-feed formula is the most convenient, but it is also the most expensive. Powder and concentrate are less expensive, but require more preparation. If you use powder or concentrate, you can prepare a day's worth of bottles at once and store them in the refrigerator, or you can prepare one bottle at a time.

Keep the formula and all bottle supplies clean. Some health care providers recommend sterilizing bottles and nipples for the first eight weeks of a baby's life. Ask your health care provider for his or her opinion. If you have a dishwasher, rinse the bottles in hot water before putting them in. If you wash them by hand, use hot, soapy water and a bottle brush to clean them. Wash the nipples in hot, soapy water and squeeze the water through the holes. When they are dry, store the nipples in a clean, covered container.

Giving the Bottle to the Baby

You do not have to warm a bottle before giving it to the baby. Most babies will drink bottles right from the refrigerator. If you want to warm it, do not leave it out of the refrigerator to warm; instead place it in a bowl of hot water. **Do not microwave a baby bottle**, because microwaves heat liquids unevenly—what feels like lukewarm milk could have pockets of scalding hot liquid in it.

When you give your baby a bottle, hold him or her close and keep the head higher than the body. If the baby's head is level or lower than the body, milk may seep from the back of the throat into the middle ear and can cause an ear infection.

Tip the bottle so that the nipple is filled with

milk. This prevents the baby from swallowing too much air. If the baby seems unable to get enough milk out of the bottle, check the nipple hole by tipping the bottle over the sink. The formula should come through the holes in a fine spray for one to two seconds, then in drops. Use a sterilized needle to enlarge the nipple hole if necessary. If the nipple hole seems large enough, but the formula still doesn't flow smoothly, loosen the nipple ring a little to let in some air.

Nipple holes that are too big may cause the baby to choke on a gush of formula or to gulp the bottle too quickly. If the hole is too big, you can boil the nipple to close the opening, and then reopen the hole to the proper size with a sterilized needle.

If the baby does not finish the bottle within an hour, throw it away. Bacteria that entered the bottle from the baby's mouth during the feeding will spoil the milk.

Never prop a bottle up in a baby's mouth, because the baby could choke on the milk. You should hold and cuddle a baby while bottle feeding. Body contact during feedings is essential for emotional and physical growth of a baby. When the baby is older, do not put him or her to bed with a bottle, as this practice can cause dental cavities in the baby's early teeth.

Bottle-fed babies generally want to eat every three to four hours during the first six weeks. **Do not put cereal, extra water, honey, sugar, or other solids in a baby's formula.** The baby's digestive system is not ready for anything other than formula or breastmilk for four to six months. To avoid allergic reactions, most doctors recommend not giving straight cow's milk to babies until they are more than one year old.

Lead in Drinking Water

When preparing a bottle of formula using tap water, it is a good idea to use only cold water from a faucet that has been running for a minute or so. Do not use hot or warm water because the lead that may be in the pipes is more easily dissolved by warm or hot water than cold. Most homes, including those built in the past five years, have copper water pipes that are put together with lead solder. Older homes may have pipes that are made completely of lead. By mixing formula with cold water that has been running for a minute or so you can avoid most of the lead that may be in your pipes.

The lead in tap water can cause lead poisoning in infants and children. Even small amounts of lead can cause children to have learning and reading disabilities, behavior problems, and reduced intelligence.

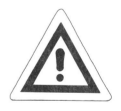

Burping

Breastfed babies should be burped after they finish one breast and before they start on the other. Some breastfed babies do not burp every time they nurse, because they don't swallow air at the breast. Bottle-fed babies can be burped halfway through a feeding and then again afterward. Babies who tend to gulp more air when feeding can be burped more frequently if necessary. **Figures 56, 57, and 58** show several positions for burping your baby.

It is normal for both breastfed and bottle-fed babies to spit up a little after a feeding. Do not be concerned, unless the baby seems ill or vomits a great deal. Spitting up after feedings is usually caused by the baby's immature digestive tract and will decrease and disappear with time.

Projectile vomiting occurs when a baby spits up milk at the end of a feeding with such force that it hits the floor or wall three or four feet away. This type of vomiting is not uncommon, but if it happens frequently the baby may need medical treatment. Tell your baby's health care provider if your baby has projectile vomiting.

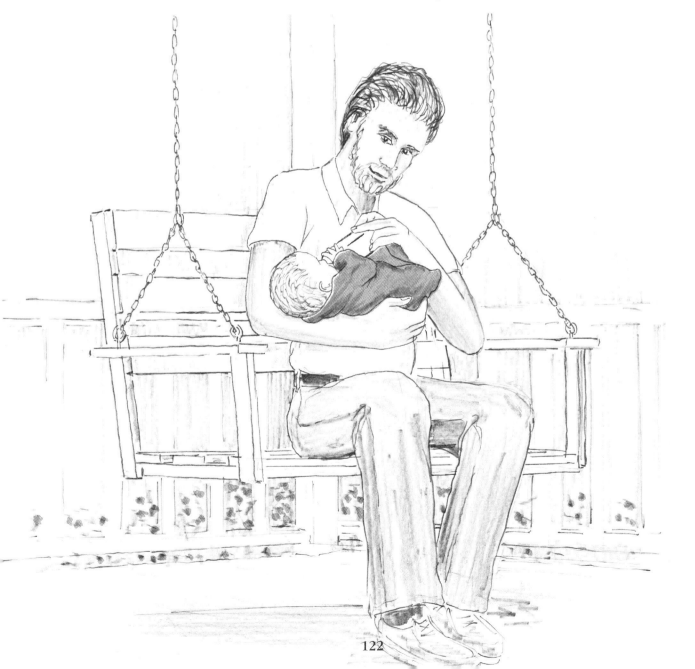

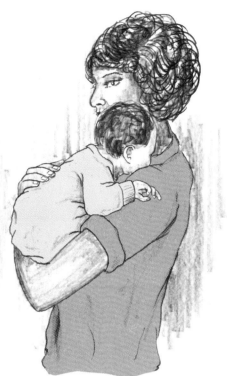

Figure 56

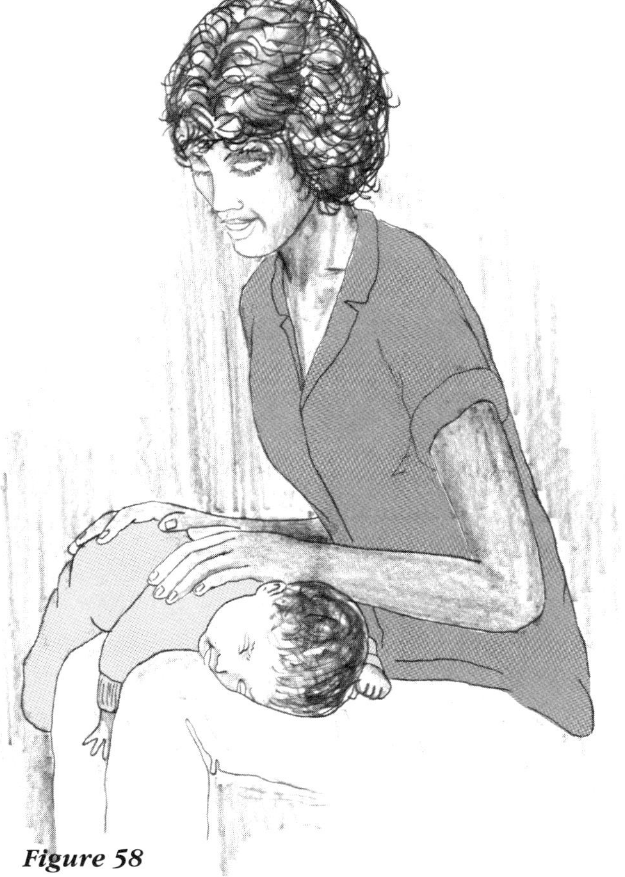

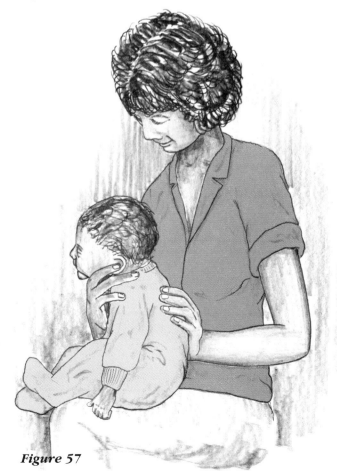

Figure 57

Figure 58

9 *Bringing Baby Home*

In this chapter, you will learn about—

- ◆ Choosing things for your baby.
- ◆ Bathing your baby.
- ◆ Diapering your baby.
- ◆ Playing with your baby.
- ◆ Adjusting to your new baby.

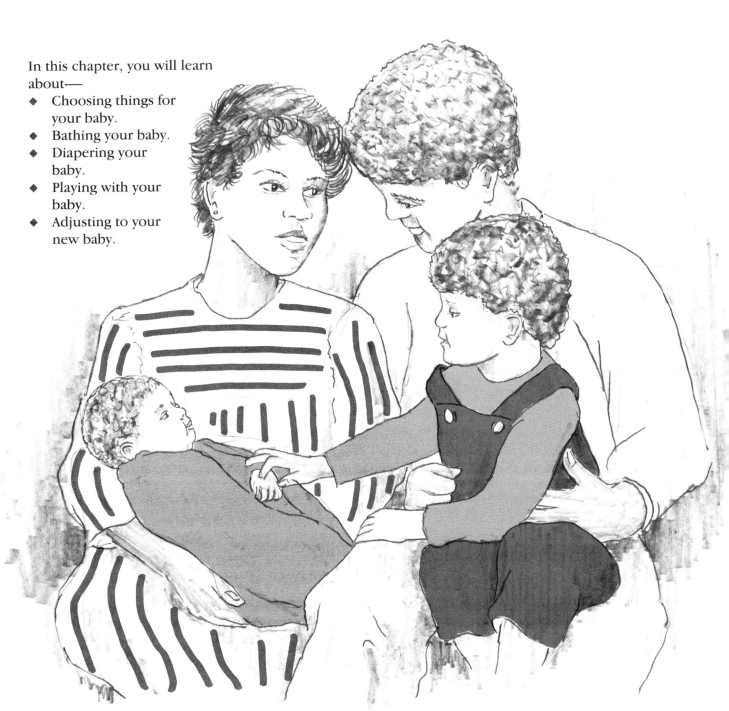

Walking over the threshold with your new baby in your arms is an exciting moment for most parents. Finally, you are home, and your family has a new member. While waiting for this moment, all kinds of thoughts probably go through your mind, especially if this is your first baby. Will you know how to hold the baby? How to diaper and bathe the baby? What will you do if the baby cries all night?

This chapter contains information about caring for your baby. It discusses what to expect in the first few weeks after birth and how to cope with the changes you will experience.

Baby Things

For being so small, babies seem to need many things! They grow so fast that it's best to stick to the basics when buying. Check with friends for hand-me-downs before you buy, and also check out second-hand stores and garage sales. Babies usually outgrow things before they wear them out. Remember to wash all items before you use them for your baby.

At first, the baby can sleep in anything with sturdy sides. A basket (such as a laundry basket) or a dresser drawer with strong sides (placed on the floor) will work as well as a cradle or bassinet. You can use a thin, plastic-covered foam pad or folded towels with a waterproof cover for a mattress. Later, your baby will need a crib. (See the section on crib safety on page 143.) The following list covers most of the basics you should try to have on hand.

Crib items
- Crib with bumper pads
- Crib sheets (four or more)
- Crib-sized waterproof mattress pads (one or two)
- Flannel-covered rubber pads to protect the mattress pad (four or more)
- Washable blankets (two) or a blanket bag or sleeping bag

Clothes
- Receiving blankets (four to six)
- T-shirts with snaps, three-month size or larger (six)
- Diapers, cloth (four dozen to six dozen) or newborn-size disposables (two boxes)
- Stretch sleepers with snaps on both legs, three-month size or larger (four or more)
- Cardigan sweater, sweatshirt, or other outer wear for cool or cold weather
- Socks or booties for cool or cold weather
- Cap for cold weather
- Sun hat

Nursery items
- Baby thermometer
- Dresser, closet, or clean box for storage of baby clothes
- Clothes hamper, basket, or box for dirty clothes
- Diaper pail with cover for cloth diapers
- Diaper bag
- Pad or blanket to change baby's diaper on
- Rocker (optional)
- Nightlight (optional)
- Wall hangings or crib mobiles, installed out of baby's reach (optional)

Toilet items
- Baby shampoo and mild soap for bathing
- Rubbing alcohol for cord care
- Zinc oxide or diaper rash ointment
- Cotton washcloths
- Cotton balls
- Plastic basin, dishpan, or tub for bathing
- Soft towels (two or three)

Health and safety items
- Auto safety seat
- Infant acetaminophen drops, for example, Tylenol
- Cool-mist vaporizer

Other items
- Infant front-pack carrier
- Bottles and nipples for bottle-fed babies

Bathing Your Baby

Most new parents worry about giving their baby a bath. However, they learn quickly that babies don't break and are very forgiving when parents are clumsy. While it is important to follow a few safety rules, you will soon find your own style of bathing your baby.

General Bathing Tips

Bathing can be a playtime for your baby, but it's a myth that all babies love their baths. Some babies enjoy their baths, while others cry all the way through them. If your baby cries, hold him or her firmly and speak gently during the bath.

Always wash from the cleanest to the dirtiest part—face first, then torso, arms, legs, and bottom. Don't pull back the foreskin of an uncircumcised infant.

Your baby doesn't need a bath every day. Keep the baby's bottom clean, and wipe the face, neck, and arms with a wet washcloth several times a day. If you do that, a bath three to four times a week is enough.

Have everything within reach before you start the bath. Once you start, it's too late to get anything else. Never leave the baby alone at bath time!

To bathe your baby, you will need—

- A washcloth.
- Mild soap.
- Water and a bathtub, pan, or sink.

Sponge Bath

Babies should be given sponge baths until the umbilical cord has fallen off (one to three weeks after birth) and the navel is completely healed. To give your baby a sponge bath—

- Undress and place the baby on a towel *(Fig. 59)*. If it's chilly, wrap the baby in another towel.
- Make sure the water temperature is correct. It should be slightly warm when you test it with your elbow.
- Wash the face with a washcloth dipped in plain water. Gently wipe each closed eye from the inner to the outer corner with the edge of the washcloth.
- Clean the outside of the ears and nose with a washcloth dipped in plain water. You don't need to clean inside the baby's ears and nose. Do not use cotton swabs at all. They can damage the ear if they are put inside too far.

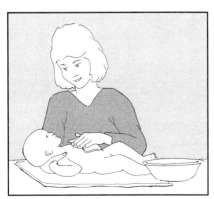

Figure 59

◆ Clean the front of the baby's body with a wet washcloth and mild soap (if you use soap). Rinse well with a washcloth dipped in plain water. Avoid wetting the navel area until the cord has healed.

◆ Turn the baby over and wash the back of the body with a wet washcloth and mild soap. Rinse well with a washcloth dipped in plain water.

◆ Wash the diaper area next. Clean the baby's genitals, using a washcloth dipped in plain water to wipe from front to back.

◆ Be sure to clean and dry all skin folds and creases carefully; they can chafe if left wet.

Tub Bath

To give your baby a tub bath—

◆ Place a towel or washcloth in the bottom of the pan, tub, or sink to keep the baby from slipping.

◆ Put about three inches of water in the tub. Test the water with your elbow. Water that is too hot can easily scald a baby's skin.

◆ Wash the face with a washcloth dipped in plain water. Gently wipe each closed eye from the inner to the outer corner with the edge of the washcloth.

◆ Clean the outside of the ears and nose with a washcloth dipped in plain water. You don't need to clean inside the baby's ears and nose. Do not use cotton swabs at all. They can damage the ear if they are put inside too far.

◆ Put the baby in the tub and hold on to him or her at all times *(Fig. 60)*. **Never leave your baby alone in the bath**—not even for a second!

◆ Wash the baby's torso, limbs, and diaper area with mild soap. Rinse well.

◆ Be sure to clean and dry all skin folds and creases carefully; they can chafe if left wet.

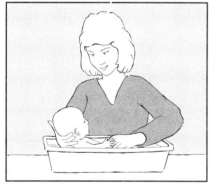
Figure 60

Washing the Hair

You can wash your baby's hair after a sponge bath or a tub bath. To wash the hair—

◆ Wrap the baby in a clean, dry towel.

◆ While you support the baby's head and neck on your arm, wet the hair with a clean washcloth and fresh water. Massage the head with a mild soap or shampoo.

◆ Rinse the baby's head with clear water, using the washcloth *(Fig. 61)*. Don't be afraid of the soft spot. It's tougher than you think. Washing a baby's hair well can help prevent cradle cap— a scaly build-up of dead skin.

◆ Pat the baby's head dry with a towel.

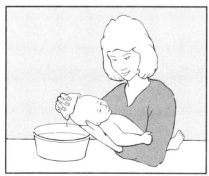
Figure 61

Massaging Your Baby

Most babies love to be touched and enjoy a soothing massage. You may use olive or vegetable oil, but it is not necessary. Massaging can be done at any time. Practice very gently at first and then use a firmer stroke as the baby gets older. Your baby will love the touch and attention. Massages also tend to bond both of the parents and the baby closer together.

Diapering

You will have to decide whether to use disposable diapers, cloth diapers you launder at home, or cloth diapers provided by a diaper service. There is a new brand of biodegradable disposable diapers now. There are advantages and disadvantages to each option:

Disposable diapers—
- Are convenient, especially when traveling.
- Save the work of laundering.
- Eliminate the need for plastic pants.
  but
- They are expensive.
- They may cause diaper rash because the outer plastic layer decreases circulation.

Home-laundered cloth diapers—
- Are the most economical.
- Have many other uses.
- May cause fewer rashes than disposables depending on the washing method used.
  but
- They require the most work.
- They can be inconvenient when you are traveling.

Diaper service diapers—
- Are more economical than disposables.
- Cause fewer diaper rashes.
- Are less work than home-laundered diapers.
  but
- They might not be accessible.
- They are more expensive to use than home-laundered diapers.

Whatever type of diapers you decide to use, for the first few months you will need 70 to 90 diapers a week. If you are using cloth diapers, you will also need rubber pants and diaper pins.

Some soaps and detergents are less irritating than others. If you are environmentally conscious, consider using biodegradable soaps or natural soaps.

You should not use baby powder, lotion, or disposable wipes on a newborn's skin. Powder may cake in the creases of the baby's legs and buttocks. Powder shaken on the baby may be inhaled and irritate the lungs. Lotion can clog pores. Disposable wipes have alcohol and other chemicals that can dry the skin.

Always keep a hand on the baby when changing the diaper. Even newborns can roll over.

Create a permanent changing place in your home where you have available all the supplies you will need:
- Water and washcloth
- Diaper pins
- Diapers
- Diaper ointment, if needed
- Cotton balls
- Alcohol for cord care

Environmental note: Whatever kind of diaper you use will have some impact on the environment. Disposable diapers are discarded after use and become part of the solid waste problem. They are not completely biodegradable. Cloth diapers have to be washed, use water and energy, and create sewage that must be treated. Strong detergents used in washing diapers may pollute the environment. If you are concerned about the environmental impact of diapers, continue to educate yourself and choose the method that seems best to you.

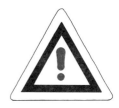

Diaper Rash

If your baby gets a diaper rash—
- Change the diaper frequently.
- Wash the affected area with warm water and pat dry to prevent further irritation.
- Expose the area to air or indirect sunlight to help the rash heal.
- Apply zinc oxide or other diaper rash ointment as recommended by your health care provider.
- If the condition continues, contact your health care provider.

Cord Care

The umbilical cord stump will fall off in 10 days to three weeks. While the cord stump is attached, when you change the diaper, clean the area around the navel with a cotton ball soaked in alcohol. If the cord becomes infected (as indicated by foul odor, discharge, or redness), contact your health care provider.

Circumcision Care

If your baby was circumcised, follow your health care provider's directions for caring for the circumcision. If there is discharge or bleeding, or if the baby seems to be in pain, call your health care provider.

Playing With Your Baby

Babies need our touch, the sight of our faces, and the sound of our voices. By playing with your baby during feeding, bathing, and diaper times, as well as during special playtimes, you are stimulating all of the baby's senses and helping him or her to grow and develop. It does not take fancy equipment, flashcards, or expertise to play with a baby. What babies need is frequent interaction with those around them. Babies learn about themselves and the world around them as they play by themselves and with others.

Babies look at objects and follow them as they move. Try holding a red apple about a foot away from the baby and moving it back and forth. Taking the baby from room to room with you visually stimulates the baby more than if you

keep him or her in one place all the time. At two or three months of age, babies begin to notice their hands, bringing them closer to their face and sometimes smacking themselves in the nose.

Babies need to have someone to talk and sing to them. When your baby is awake, you also can play the radio, stereo, or a music box softly.

Touch is very important for babies. They need to be held close, cuddled, stroked, and hugged. Being rocked and moved around is also important and will often calm a cranky infant. **You cannot spoil your baby by holding him or her.**

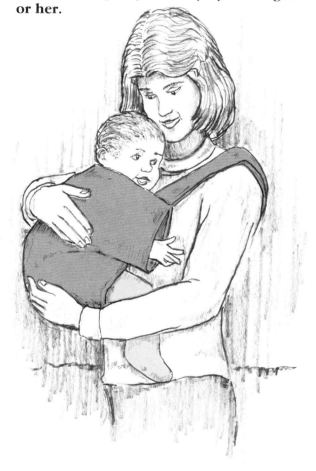

Babies love soft toys they can grasp and hold. Toys should be large enough that the baby can't swallow them, and they should have smooth, rounded edges and no small parts that can fall off. Introduce one or two toys at a time, and change them frequently. Household objects are best: cloths of different textures, wooden spoons, and large balls of wadded paper are examples of items that will do just fine for your baby.

Adjusting to the Baby

Adjusting to a new baby in the house, especially a first baby, is probably the biggest change most people ever undergo. The physical and emotional changes the mother experiences after the baby is born, role changes for both parents, and the 24-hour demands of a newborn make this a stressful, if joyful, period. While you may expect perfection, reality sets in more often than you might wish.

Don't expect to return to your normal size the instant the baby is born. It takes from six weeks to six months to return to your prepregnancy size. Stringent dieting is not recommended in the first weeks after birth because you need energy to recover from the demands of pregnancy and birth. **If you are breastfeeding, you should not diet at all.** Make sure you eat a well-balanced diet that emphasizes fresh fruits and vegetables, protein, and adequate fluids. It will help you regain your energy while you lose weight slowly.

Adding a mild exercise program will also help you to get back in shape. Start with gentle toning exercises such as the ones you have learned in this course. See your health care provider for advice and suggestions before you resume exercise.

It is very common for new mothers to have "postpartum blues" in the first three to five days after the baby is born. This period is often characterized by moodiness, crying, depression, and fatigue. Usually these feelings fade as your hormones begin to settle down. If after a few weeks these feelings still persist, or if you feel unable to care for yourself or your baby, you should contact your health care provider. Getting the rest you need, eating well, practicing relaxation and visualization exercises, and receiving support from your family and/or friends can decrease postpartum blues.

One of the most difficult aspects of new-baby care is the inability to predict anything. Sometimes it is impossible to know when you will be able to take a shower, eat a meal sitting down, or talk with your partner. Nothing completely prepares first parents for the newborn period. Everything is totally new and different, and it happens 24 hours a day. Sometimes you may be angry at your baby for disrupting you all the time. This is normal. You still love your baby but are upset with the present situation. If, however, you feel that you might hurt your baby or feel unable to care for him or her, you should call someone to help you right away, such as a friend, a relative, or your local social service agency.

Already tired from the demands of labor, a new mother must care for a baby who makes demands day and night. Both mothers and fathers need extra rest in the postpartum period, but this is likely to take place in spurts rather than in eight-hour stretches.

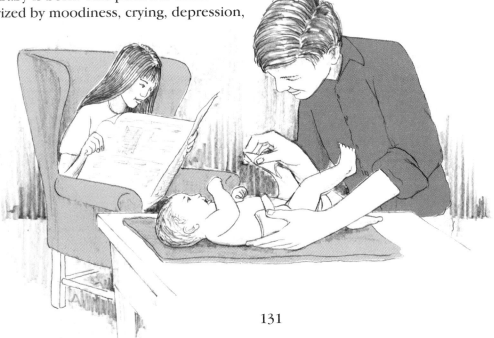

The New Baby
A Fantasy... A Reality

A Fantasy

Ruffles, soft music, cherubic sleeping infant. Small, fragrant being awakens every four hours... exactly. Eats well, burps on schedule, returns to peaceful slumber.

Smiling friends... helpful (but not too helpful) relatives.

Fitting back into size nine clothes the first day home.

A flat belly.

Husband comes home after work to sparkling house, delicious hot meal. Enjoys noticing wife in sexy black negligee holding sweet-smelling, cooing infant in one hand, soda for him in the other.

A Reality

Husband goes off to work without breakfast since toaster is lost under dirty dishes.

Wife decides it is not worthwhile to remove rumpled terry robe since size nine clothes fit left leg only.

Hair uncombed, must plan ahead to take shower.

Wife's bottom hurts... no need for sexy black negligee.

Baby crying, demanding, unaware his diaper has just been changed.

Relatives bossy, too many visitors.

Always, perpetually, and forever **tired**.

Husband comes home from work, sees chaos, leaves for McDonald's.

From Pincus, Linda. "Reality Versus Fantasy: Preparing Parents for the Postpartum Period." *Genesis* 5:16, June/July 1983.

Tips for Coping

Here are some suggestions for how to cope in the first few weeks after you bring your baby home:

- **Get help and support from others**—Ask for help when you need it—from your partner, relatives, and friends. Friends can bring a casserole or help to care for an older child. Your family or friends can help with the cleaning or the cooking. As parents, you should be spending your time caring for and getting to know your baby—that's the most important thing you can do in the postpartum period.

- **Relax your standards**—Newborns don't need a spotless house—they aren't crawling yet. Relax your standards of housework during this period.

- **Communicate**—New parents should let each other know when something is bothering them and try to resolve it. Even though you may feel that communicating with your partner is just one more thing in your hectic day, it is very important to make time for each other to keep from growing apart or storing up grievances.

- **Nap**—Rest often, and nap whenever you can. You need to make up for lost sleep. Sleep when the baby sleeps, unplug the phone, put a "Do Not Disturb" sign on the door. Going to bed earlier also will help.

- **Eat well**—Good nutrition is important. It will help you to regain your strength and to heal from the birth.

- **Relax and visualize**—The skills you learned in Chapters 4 and 6 can be used to help you relax. In addition, babies are sensitive to their parents' moods, so if you can be calm, you may find your baby calming down too. Relaxation will have a positive effect on you and all of those around you.

- **Take time out**—New parents need time away—together and alone—even if it's just an hour between feedings to take a walk, go to the grocery store, or sit at a cafe. These are all ways of taking a break. Finding a babysitter that you trust may take time, but it is worth it. Sometimes you may be able to save costs by trading off babysitting with other parents. Many neighborhoods and military housing units have established baby-sitting co-ops that allow new parents an opportunity to take some time for themselves.

Role Changes

Changing from being partners to being parents too requires a major adjustment. Even if you have prepared carefully, there will be surprises. You may think, "I'm just a child myself," even if you are in your twenties or thirties. It is important to sort out what you can realistically expect from yourself and each other in the first few weeks. If you haven't done the Family Roles exercise on pages 33 and 34, do it now, or review what you did earlier. Talk about what you expect from each other and from your first days at home with the baby.

Brothers and Sisters

Brothers and sisters should be introduced to the new baby as soon as possible. Allow them, with careful supervision, to touch or hold the baby. It is normal for older children to be jealous of the time that parents spend with this new member of the family. They may wonder whether their parents still love them. For reassurance, they need special time alone with both parents. Sometimes younger children do babyish things, such as sucking their thumbs, crying more, or asking for diapers or bottles. They may need extra attention or some time alone with mother and/or father. Help them see that they are more grown-up than the new baby and can do more exciting things.

Young children should not be left alone with a new baby because they cannot understand the need for safety. Parents can encourage them to help in whatever way they can (bringing diapers, patting the baby, helping with the bath), but an adult should always be present.

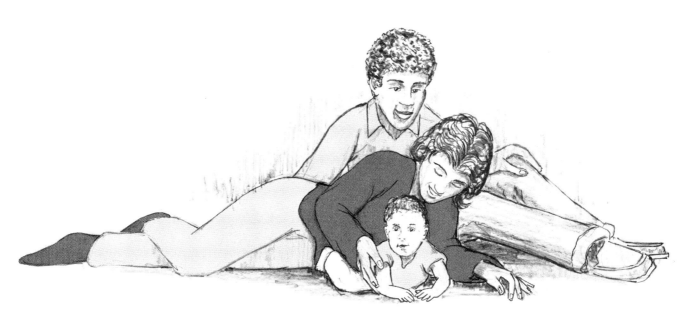

Crying and Sleeping

Babies communicate most often by crying. Reasons a baby cries include—

◆ Hunger.
◆ Loneliness.
◆ Being tired, wet, or soiled.
◆ Being in one position too long.
◆ Boredom.

It is your job to figure out the cause of the crying and to do something about it. Most of the time you can. No baby should be left to cry for a long time without someone trying to soothe and comfort him or her. However, there may be occasions when you have done everything you know how, and the baby is still crying. If this happens, it is fine to take a break. Put the baby in the crib or give the baby to someone else to take care of before trying again to see what's wrong.

It is very important for you to know that **you cannot spoil a baby**. Babies whose needs are responded to quickly and consistently in the first year of life build up a sense of trust. They are usually less fussy later in the first year if their needs have been met in the early months.

There are many ways to soothe a crying baby. For example, you can—

◆ Pick the baby up and hold him or her close.
◆ Rock the baby in a comfortable rocking chair.
◆ Try switching positions, perhaps putting the baby over your shoulder so the stomach is resting on the top of your shoulder.

◆ Wrap (swaddle) the baby in a blanket snugly. Some infants feel more secure this way.
◆ Put the baby in a front-pack next to your chest and walk around. You can even get some work done this way.
◆ Lay the baby across your knees and move your knees up and down. This helps many parents get through dinner.
◆ Take the baby out for a ride in the stroller or in the car. Day or night, the distraction will help you as well as the baby.

Most of the concerns parents have about their baby's sleeping habits revolve around the baby's ability to sleep through the night. It is normal for babies to wake up two or three times during the night in the first six weeks to three months. Someone will very likely advise you to give the baby cereal as a way to induce a longer sleeping period, but don't do it. The baby's body cannot digest solids yet. Your health care provider will tell you when your baby is developed enough to handle solids.

Babies can be put in a crib as soon as they are brought home. For the first few weeks, you may wish to have your baby sleep nearby in a bassinet. Babies differ in how much sleep they need—12 to 20 hours a day. They will naturally get the amount they need. It is not necessary, and in fact is inadvisable, to be extra quiet around a sleeping baby. Most will sleep through anything, and it is best to get them used to normal household noise.

10 *Infant Health and Safety*

In this chapter, you will learn about—

◆ Choosing your baby's health care provider.
◆ Well-baby care.
◆ Taking steps to make your baby safe.
◆ Emergencies and how to respond to them.

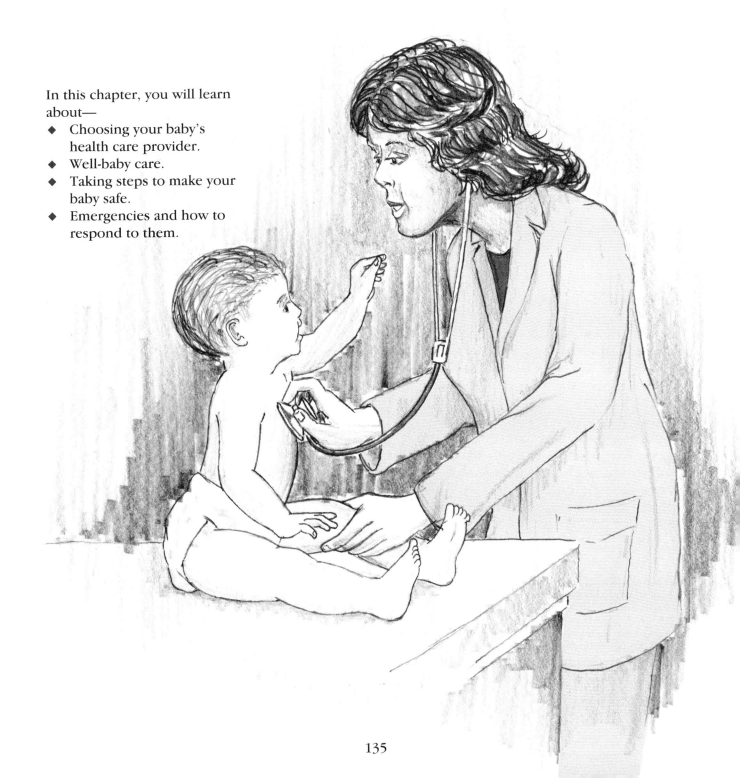

One of your most important jobs as a parent is to ensure your baby's health and safety. This includes finding a health care provider for your baby, knowing when to take your baby to the provider, knowing when your baby is sick, knowing how to care for a sick baby, and taking steps to make sure that your baby is safe. This chapter discusses all of these topics.

Baby's Health Care Provider

You should have a health care provider for your baby, even before the baby is born. If you will be using a military clinic or a public health clinic, you may be assigned to a health care provider. Otherwise you will choose your baby's provider. In either case, you will probably want to get answers to some or all of the following questions:

- Is the provider's office conveniently located, so that you can travel there easily?
- Is the provider available for telephone advice?
- With what hospital does the provider have privileges?
- Do you feel comfortable with and trust the provider?
- Do you feel that the provider will take the time to answer questions or help you make the adjustment to parenthood?
- How does the provider feel about issues important to you, such as breastfeeding or going back to work?
- Does the provider practice alone, or are there others in the practice?
- Does your insurance cover this provider?

If your health care provider has privileges in the hospital where your baby is born, he or she will examine the baby there before the baby is discharged. If not, the hospital will assign a provider to examine your baby. Most providers also want to see a baby in their office when the baby is two weeks old, or even sooner if the baby was discharged early or has any special problems. In addition, the baby should see the provider many times in the first year—both for well-baby checkups and for any problems that may occur.

Before you leave the hospital, you should know where the provider's office is and what telephone number to call if you have questions in the first two weeks.

Well-Baby Care and Immunizations

For the first few years, you will visit your baby's health care provider so that the provider can monitor your baby's growth and development and give your baby immunizations. A baby usually has a checkup when he or she is two weeks old and then every four to eight weeks thereafter for the first year. Often the most important part of the baby's checkup is your conversation with the health care provider. You will probably have many questions and concerns in the first few weeks. It is helpful to talk these over with the health care provider. Find out if there is an advice nurse or a specific time for telephone calls so that you can call when you have concerns between visits. It is always a good idea to write down your questions and observations before calling so that they are easier to remember.

It is very important that you have your baby immunized according to schedule in the early years. Babies up to a year old are at risk for developing serious complications from early childhood diseases and should be protected. Also, keep your own record of well-baby visits and immunizations (including the dates) in case you move or change providers. (See the "Immunization Record," Appendix H). Update the record each time the baby is seen. Child care providers and schools require proof that a child has been properly immunized.

Immunization Schedule	
Age	**Immunization**
2 months	Diphtheria-pertussis-tetanus (DPT) vaccine, polio vaccine, Hemophilus type b conjugate vaccine (Hib vaccine)*
4 months	DPT vaccine, polio vaccine, Hib vaccine
6 months	DPT vaccine, Hib vaccine
12 months	TB (tuberculosis) test
15 months	Measles, mumps, rubella (MMR) vaccine, Hib vaccine
16–24 months	DPT vaccine, polio vaccine
4–6 years	DPT vaccine, polio vaccine
11–12 years	MMR vaccine
12–16 years	Tetanus-diphtheria (TD) vaccine
Every 10 years thereafter	TD vaccine

* Hib vaccine protects infants and children from meningitis, pneumonia, epiglottitis (a severe form of croup), and other serious infections.

Well-Baby Visits

In a well-baby visit, the health care provider will check your baby's growth (height, weight, and head circumference). The provider will also check the baby's sight and hearing and do a physical exam that includes testing the baby's normal reflexes. He or she will ask you questions about your baby's activities and give you an idea of what to expect before your next visit. This is a good time for you to ask questions and discuss anything that may be worrying you.

Sick Babies

Despite everything you do, babies sometimes get sick. Usually you will know that your baby is sick because of the way he or she looks and behaves. If you are at all concerned about your baby's health, it is best to call your health care provider. Try to note all the differences you see in your baby's behavior. Here are some signs and symptoms of illness for which you should call your health care provider:

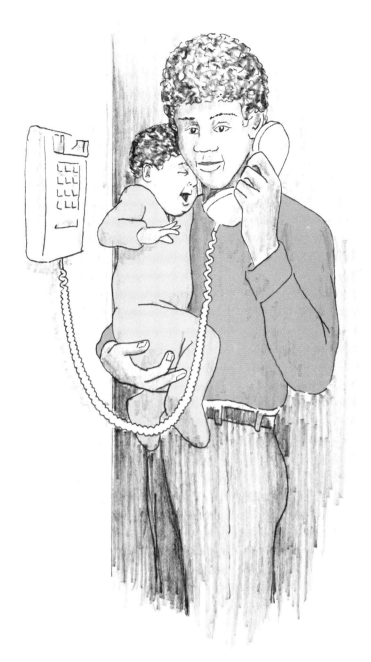

- ◆ Fever
- ◆ Vomiting
- ◆ Diarrhea
- ◆ Coughing
- ◆ Difficulty breathing
- ◆ Excessive crying
- ◆ Lethargy
- ◆ Blood in the urine or stool
- ◆ Decreased urination (fewer than six wet diapers a day)
- ◆ Changes in behavior (such as increased irritability, decreased activity, or more crying than usual)
- ◆ Pulling at an ear
- ◆ Loss of appetite

Fever

Even mild fevers in the first months of the baby's life should be reported to the health care provider. You should know how to take your baby's temperature and always have a thermometer in the house. Always contact the health care provider in the early months before you give any medication for a fever. **Never give aspirin to a baby or child with a fever.** Some studies have shown that use of aspirin has been associated with a very serious illness called Reye's syndrome.

Taking the Temperature

There are two ways to take a baby's temperature. You can put the thermometer under the baby's arm or you can put it in the baby's rectum.

To take a baby's temperature under the arm—

◆ Use a rectal or oral thermometer *(Fig. 62)*.

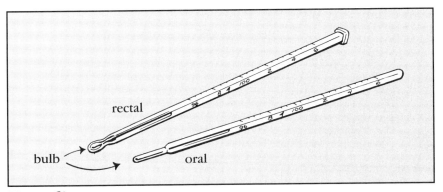

Figure 62

◆ Shake the mercury level down to below 96 degrees fahrenheit or 36 degrees celsius.
◆ Put the bulb under the baby's armpit and hold the baby's arm close to his or her body for five minutes *(Fig. 63)*.
◆ Read the thermometer.
◆ Clean the thermometer with soapy, warm water, and store it in its case.
◆ Wash your hands.
◆ Write down the baby's temperature. The normal temperature for a baby is 97.6–99.6 degrees fahrenheit or 36.4–37.6 degrees celsius.

To take baby's rectal temperature—

◆ Use a rectal thermometer only *(Fig. 62)*.
◆ Shake the mercury down to below 96 degrees fahrenheit or 36 degrees celsius.
◆ Lubricate the bulb of the thermometer with petroleum jelly.
◆ Lay the baby across your lap, stomach down. Gently insert the bulb no more than one inch into the baby's rectum. Keep your hands against the baby's bottom to prevent injury in case he or she wiggles *(Fig. 64)*.
◆ Take the thermometer out after three minutes.
◆ Wipe off the thermometer and read it.
◆ Clean the thermometer with soapy, warm water, and store it in its case.
◆ Wash your hands.
◆ Write down the baby's temperature. The normal temperature for a baby is 97.6–99.6 degrees fahrenheit or 36.4–37.6 degrees celsius.

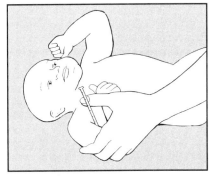

Figure 63

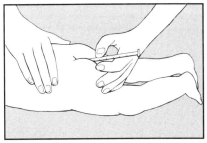

Figure 64

Common Illnesses

Almost all babies become ill at some time, so you should know how to deal with the most common illnesses. These include—

♦ **Vomiting**—Most babies spit up some of their feedings some of the time. Vomiting, however, is more forceful, with most of the stomach contents coming up. If vomiting occurs more than once in 24 hours, call the health care provider.

♦ **Diarrhea**—If an infant has more than one very loose or watery stool in a day, call the health care provider. Infants can become dehydrated very easily from diarrhea, and the fluids lost have to be replaced. Signs of dehydration include dry mouth, sunken soft spots on the head, drowsiness, lack of energy, dry skin, decreased urination (fewer than six wet diapers a day), and fever.

♦ **Colds**—Signs of a cold include a runny or stopped-up nose; red, watery eyes; a dry cough; breathing difficulty due to a stuffy nose; listlessness or loss of appetite; and sometimes a fever. There is no medicine that cures a cold. Colds are best treated by making the baby more comfortable. To make the infant more comfortable, use a cool-water humidifier, place the infant on his or her side for sleeping, and raise the head of the crib by placing a pillow or books under the mattress (this helps drain the mucus). If an infant develops a fever, cries a lot, has any difficulty breathing, or coughs up green or gray sputum, call the health care provider without delay.

♦ **Ear infections**—Middle-ear infections are common in young children. They may occur in conjunction with, or after, a cold. Children with middle-ear infections may be very fussy, wake up in the night screaming, and rub or pull at their ears. Your health care provider will usually prescribe antibiotics for the infection and acetaminophen (Tylenol) for pain relief.

Keeping Your Baby Safe

Having a baby around requires a very careful eye. One of the greatest threats to healthy babies is injury, which can cause serious harm or even death. You have to be alert constantly to any situation or anything that could injure your baby. You should take steps to create a safe environment for your baby.

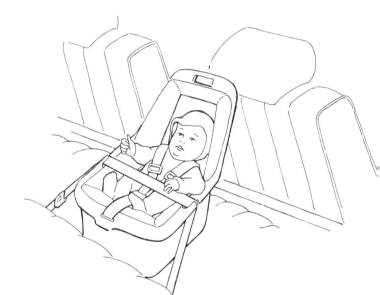

Safety in the Car

One of the most important things you can do to make your baby safe is to get an approved car safety seat and use it properly every time your baby rides in a motor vehicle. You should begin now, before your baby is born, to figure out where you will get a car safety seat, which model is best for you, and which will fit in your car. You will need it right away if you plan to take your baby home from the hospital in a car.

One of the most important reasons to use a safety seat is to protect your child from being severely injured or even killed in a car crash. Another reason is that it is now a law in every state in the United States and in many foreign countries. Most hospitals will not allow you to take your newborn home unless you have a safety seat. Whether you are in the United States or abroad, and whether it is a law or not, it is absolutely necessary to use a safety seat to protect your baby.

Safety Seats

What are some of the reasons you should always use a safety seat for your child?

_____

_____

_____

_____

_____

What are some of the reasons some people don't use safety seats for their child?

_____

_____

_____

_____

_____

There are many foolish reasons why people do not use a safety seat for their baby. For example, some people believe that their baby is safer in their arms when they are riding in a car. Nothing could be farther from the truth. A baby being held in an adult's arms could be crushed by the adult during a crash, or the baby could be thrown out of the adult's grasp, into the windshield, or out through the window. See "Myths and Facts About Safety Seats" in Appendix I for other examples.

Safety seats must be used from the time your baby first rides in a car until he or she weighs about 40 pounds or is about four years old. After that, the child should use either a safety belt or a booster seat. **Restraints must be used on every ride.** Remember, you should always buckle up too.

If a safety seat is involved in a crash, don't use it again. The seat may be damaged, even if it looks okay to you. After a crash, the safety belts of the car also should be checked. They might have been damaged and need replacement.

There are three different types of safety seats:

◆ The **infant model** is for infants up to about one year old and up to 20 pounds. Infant seats must always face backward toward the rear of the vehicle and be in a semireclined position. Infants fit best in this type of seat.

◆ The **convertible model** is for infants, toddlers, and preschoolers up to 40 pounds and about four years old. It can be used as an infant seat for babies up to 20 pounds and one year old. It faces backward in a semireclined position. As the child grows, it can be converted into a forward-facing seat, which should be upright.

◆ **Booster seats** are for children between three and eight years old (up to about 65 pounds) who have outgrown convertible seats.

Make sure you always use the manufacturer's instructions, which should be attached to the seat. If they are not there, be sure you get them before you use the seat.

Where to Get Safety Seats

You can purchase a federally approved safety seat from many retail stores and catalogs or, if you are affiliated with the military, you may obtain one on the base. Refer to the "1991 Family Shopping Guide to Car Seats" in Appendix J.

You may also rent a seat from a community loan program. Some Red Cross chapters operate a K.I.S.S. (Kids in Safety Seats) program that rents infant seats at a very low cost. Some chapters have the same type of program for toddlers as well. If you borrow a seat or buy one second-hand, make sure that it still has the manufacturer's instructions with it. Ask if it has ever been in a crash, even a minor collision. If it has, don't use it. Find out how old the seat is. If the label has a manufacture date earlier than 1981, the seat does not meet the current standards for crash protection. Do not use the seat. In addition, some seats manufactured after 1981 have experienced safety problems and have been recalled by the manufacturer. Be sure to find out as much information as you can about the seat you have. To find out more information, call the U.S. Department of Transportation Safety Seat Hotline at 1–800–424–9393 or your local Transportation or Motor Vehicle safety office.

Safety at Home

Injuries are a leading cause of death to children, but most could be prevented if everyone followed general safety rules. Although some of the safety tips listed below are for older children, they are included so that you can provide a safe environment for your baby right from the start.

Baths

◆ Turn the thermostat on your hot water heater down to below 120 degrees fahrenheit or 49 degrees celsius.
◆ Always check the bath water temperature with your elbow to avoid burning the baby.
◆ Keep one hand on the baby at all times in the bath. **Never leave the baby alone in the bath.**

Falls

◆ Never turn your back on a baby who is on a table, bed, or chair.
◆ Always keep the crib rails up.
◆ If interrupted when caring for your baby, put the baby in the crib, under your arm, or on the floor.

- Never leave the baby unattended in an infant seat on a table or counter.
- Hold on to the handrail when you carry the baby down the stairs.
- Keep stairways clear of objects that could cause you to fall while you are holding the baby.

Burns

- Put screens around hot radiators, floor furnaces, stoves, or kerosene heaters.
- Don't smoke or let care givers smoke when they are around your baby.
- Don't hold your baby and drink a hot beverage at the same time.
- Don't leave a filled coffee or tea cup near a table edge where it could be pulled down or knocked over.
- Be sure that foods, bottles, and bath water are not too hot.
- Do not heat baby food or bottles in a microwave oven.
- Do not try to cook and hold the baby at the same time.
- Make sure the electric cords of irons, coffee makers, and other hot appliances are not dangling from counters.

Crib, Bassinet, Carriage, and Playpen

- All paint on anything you put your baby in must be lead-free. (An old crib, bassinet, carriage, or playpen should be stripped of its paint and painted with lead-free enamel paint—check the labels. This should not be done by a pregnant woman.)
- The space between crib and playpen slats should be no more than 2–3/8 inches. Other openings, such as decorative cutouts, should be avoided.
- Wood surfaces should be smooth and splinter-free.
- The crib mattress should fit snugly. You shouldn't be able to get more than two fingers between the mattress and the crib side.
- When the mattress is in the crib, the crib side in the raised position should be at least 20 inches above the mattress surface.
- Use bumper pads until the baby learns to pull to a standing position.

- Remove plastic wrap from the mattress (children can suffocate).
- Don't use a pillow.
- Don't put a harness or straps on the baby in the crib.
- Don't hang any toy or mobile across the crib if there is any chance the baby could touch it with any part of his or her body.

Other

- Select toys that are too large to swallow, too tough to break, and do not have any small breakable parts or sharp edges or points.
- Keep pins, buttons, coins, and plastic bags out of the baby's reach.
- Never put anything—except what is all right for a baby to eat or drink—in a baby bottle, baby food jar, or dish.
- Never put a loop of ribbon or cord around the baby's neck to hold a pacifier, or for any other reason.
- Do not put necklaces or rings on the baby. It's too easy for the baby to swallow them.
- When the baby is asleep or unsupervised, take all toys and small objects out of the crib or playpen.
- Keep the telephone numbers of the baby's health care provider, the hospital, the emergency medical service system, and the poison control center posted next to your telephone.
- Install smoke detectors if you do not already have them. Keep a small fire extinguisher in the kitchen out of the children's reach.
- Never leave a bottle propped up for your baby to drink.

Emergencies

No matter how careful you are, injuries and illnesses can occur. You should know what to do in case of an emergency. Taking an American Red Cross Infant and Child CPR course or Standard First Aid course is highly recommended to increase your confidence in knowing how to care for your child in an emergency situation. You should post the Instructions for Emergency Telephone Calls (Appendix K) near your telephone and make sure that every member of the family and any other care giver knows they are there.

When to Call the EMS System

Call the emergency medical services (EMS) system if—

◆ The baby is not breathing or is experiencing difficulty breathing. (The baby may be having difficulty breathing if the baby's breathing appears labored; if the baby's general skin color is pale, blue, or grayish, or the lips and fingernails are bluish or gray; or if the baby is difficult to wake up).

◆ The baby is unconscious (you are unable to wake up the baby, even if he or she is breathing).

◆ The baby is choking.

◆ The baby has no pulse.

◆ The baby is bleeding severely.

◆ The baby is burned.

Appendixes L and M give instructions on what to do if your infant is choking and how to do rescue breathing. While these are not a substitute for taking a CPR course, it is a good reminder of what you should do if your baby is choking or stops breathing.

11 Planning Ahead

In this chapter, you will learn—
- How to arrange for maternity leave.
- How to ease your transition back to work and the baby's transition to a child care situation.
- How to share responsibility for home and baby care.
- How to stay healthy.
- How to stay close to your partner while juggling work and home responsibilities.
- About family planning and contraception.

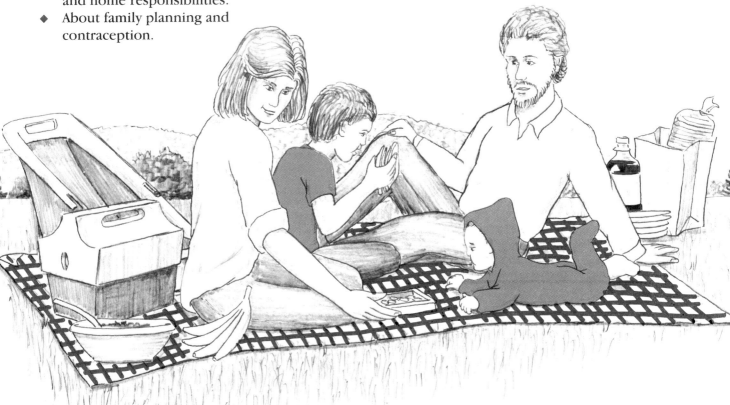

Planning Ahead

This chapter discusses some of the issues that arise when a mother returns to work after the birth of a child. It covers some of the problems many parents face in trying to balance attention to home and work responsibilities. It gives tips to parents on how to take care of themselves and the baby when they both work.

The chapter also covers family planning and methods of birth control, so you and your partner can discuss these subjects frankly and realistically.

Going Back to Work

For women who worked before they became pregnant, deciding whether or not to return to work after the baby is born may be simple in practical terms. Many families depend on two paychecks to meet their living expenses. Because of that, more women than ever before are returning to work soon after their babies are born. Some women just like to work and don't want to stop after the baby is born.

A new mother who returns to work for whatever reason can expect the transition to be complicated. Although she may welcome the return to work life, leaving a new baby with another care giver is never easy. And trying to keep on top of the demands of a job, in addition to the demands of a newborn, is a big task. This chapter offers some suggestions on ways to make the return to work a little easier.

If you work now and plan to return to work after the baby is born, you may find yourself patching together leave without pay, vacation leave, and sick or disability leave to have a few weeks or months at home with your newborn. Whether you work in a job with very limited benefits or in one with generous benefits, you should find out now how much leave you will be able to take.

When you inform your employer that you are pregnant, be prepared to say how long you expect to work before the baby is born and how long you wish to be on maternity leave. Get specific information on your employer's policy on maternity leave and a clear statement about your ability to return to work and about your benefits, such as pay and seniority.

Fathers who want to stay home for a while with their new baby can follow the same tips, but

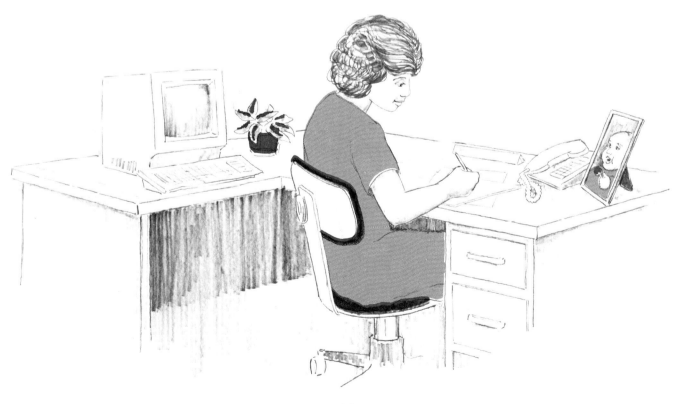

Financial Costs and Benefits of Working

Benefits of Working
(Monthly Amount You Receive)

Salary (net) $ _____

Health insurance   _____

Child care tax deduction   _____

A. Total Benefits: $ _____

Costs of Working
(Monthly Amount You Pay)

Child care $ _____

Wardrobe for work   _____

Commuting   _____

Meals out at restaurants   _____

Additional taxes   _____

Relying on carryout or convenience foods rather than home cooking   _____

Other costs:

_____   _____

_____   _____

_____   _____

_____   _____

B. Total Costs: $ _____

Your total benefits (A) $ _____
minus
Your total costs (B)   − $ _____
equals
Your financial gain (or loss) if you work $ _____

they should be prepared for less support from their employer. Those who do get time off, however, will enjoy some very special time with the new member of their family.

Working: Costs and Benefits

If you feel uncertain whether going back to work is something you want to do, fill in the Financial Costs and Benefits of Working chart on page 147. If the costs of working come close to the income and other benefits you will bring in, you may find that by tightening your budget a little, you are able to come out ahead financially and stay home with your baby, if that is what you want to do.

In addition to the financial considerations, you should take into account how you feel about your job and how your taking time off will affect your career, earnings, and social security benefits in the future. If something should happen to your spouse and you are not working, do you have enough savings or life insurance to tide you over until you are able to reenter the work force? Other considerations include the availability of good child care, your philosophy of parenting, the needs of the child, and any other personal feelings related to work and home.

How to Ease the Transition Back to Work

Making the transition back to work involves emotional as well as practical adjustments. Your daily routine will become more complicated as you juggle your responsibilities to the baby, to your home, and to your job. You will also have to get accustomed to the way it feels to leave your baby in someone else's care while you are at work.

Once you have found a child care provider you trust, you should consider working part-time for a week or two, to ease yourself back into working and the baby into his or her relationship with the care giver. It may help to begin your first week back at work on a Wednesday or Thursday so that you work a few days and then have the weekend to recover before you work a full week. In any case, it is a good idea for you to spend some time together with the baby and the care giver before you leave the baby with the care giver. This way, you can give the care giver

specific information about caring for the baby.

Most working parents find it is very difficult to perform on their jobs as they did before their baby was born, or to have enough energy left at the end of the day to take care of the baby. You should practice saving some energy for the end of the day so that your baby and your relationship with your partner are not short-changed. Try to find ways to get jobs done more easily. Do something relaxing at your lunch hour, and limit the number of your social engagements. Try to take time during the day to use the visualization and relaxation skills you learned in this course to help you have more energy and feel better. When you get home, learn to accept a less-than-spotless house and less-complicated meals.

It's very important to find ways to save time and energy for your baby so you will feel good about yourself as a parent. If you don't, you may try to compensate by overstimulating the baby. Babies need calm, centered, loving attention from their parents. Some of the most enjoyable times you will spend with your baby are those spontaneous moments when the baby looks at you and laughs or reaches for a toy for the first time. You will miss these moments if you are constantly rushed. Take the time to enjoy your baby. He or she will be crawling, then walking, and then going to school before you know it.

Breastfeeding and Working

If you want to continue to breastfeed after you return to work, start giving your baby a bottle when he or she is between three and six weeks old. If you start earlier than this, the baby may become confused and have difficulty at the breast. If you start later than six weeks, the baby may refuse to take milk from any nipple other than yours.

Have someone give the bottle to the baby when he or she is not frantically hungry—between feedings is best at first. Most babies associate their mother's scent and sound with nursing and refuse to take a bottle from her. She may even have to leave the room since the baby will be aware she is present and will not want to take the bottle. This is an ideal opportunity for the baby's father to take a larger role in the baby's feedings. Try different kinds of nipples until you find one the baby will accept. The shape of a contoured (orthodontic) nipple conforms more closely to that of the human nipple.

If you plan to leave your own milk for the child care provider to feed to your baby, you will need to learn how to express milk while you are at work. Start expressing milk before you return to work so that you don't have to learn "on the job." A good time to start is in the morning after the first feeding.

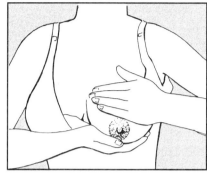

Figure 65

You should know how to express milk even if you aren't returning to work. You may want to leave a bottle of breast milk if you go out and have to miss a feeding. You can express milk by hand or use a manual, battery-operated, or electric breast pump. Expressing by hand takes practice, but some women find it much easier and more convenient than using a pump.

To encourage your let-down reflex, you can look at a picture of your baby or imagine that you are cuddling him or her. You can use the visualization skills taught in Chapter 4 to help you imagine being with your baby.

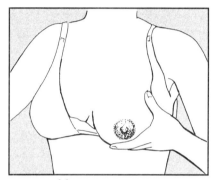

Figure 66

To express breastmilk by hand—

1. Wash you hands well and get a clean cup or bowl to catch the expressed milk. Support your left breast with the palm of your right hand. With the palm of your left hand stroke repeatedly downward on your chest as far as the areola. Massage evenly all around the breast *(Fig. 65)*.
2. Place the thumb of your left hand about halfway between the top of the breast and your nipple *(Fig. 66)*. (You may either continue to support the breast with your right hand or remove your right hand—whichever is more comfortable for you.)
3. Push your thumb down the breast toward the areola *(Fig. 67)*. As your thumb reaches the edge of the areola, press in and up and milk will squirt out *(Fig. 68)*. Do not actually touch the nipple.
4. Repeat this process on the right breast.

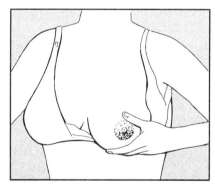

Figure 67

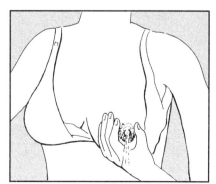

Figure 68

Electric pumps are very expensive, but they can be rented. Ask your health care provider or La Leche League representative for recommendations and sources of breast pumps in your area. You may have to work out an arrangement with your employer to use an empty office or other quiet, private space for your pumping sessions. If there is a nurse's office at your workplace, you may be able to pump there.

If there are other new mothers at your workplace, ask them if they breastfeed their babies and whether they express milk at work. Having support at work will help you in your plan to continue breastfeeding.

Most breast pumps have a built-in receptacle for the expressed milk *(Fig. 69).* Be sure that this container or any other you use is clean. You will also need a refrigerated storage place for the milk. If you do not have access to a refrigerator at work, you should bring your own cooler to work every day.

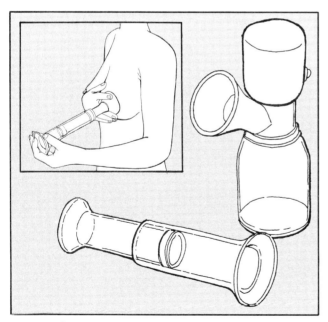

Figure 69

When you get home, label and date your breast milk and store it in your freezer, unless you intend to feed it to the baby within 24 hours. Breast milk can be stored for up to 24 hours in the refrigerator and for one month in the freezer. To thaw frozen milk, put the container holding the milk in a dish of warm, not hot, water or let

it thaw in the refrigerator. Do not thaw frozen milk in the microwave oven or on the stove.

Some mothers prefer that their baby have formula while they are at work and to nurse the baby when they are at home. All sorts of combinations of bottle feeding and breastfeeding are possible, depending on what works best for you. Your body will gradually adjust to the breastfeeding schedule you and your baby develop. Be sure you continue to eat well, rest when possible, and drink plenty of fluids to maintain your milk supply.

Taking Care of Yourself

A healthy diet and exercise are important parts of anyone's plan for feeling good. New parents often find they are so busy, tired, or stressed that they do not exercise or that they consistently make food choices based on convenience rather than nutritional value. Here are some suggestions on ways that you can make a healthy diet and exercise plan part of your life:

◆ Cook meals ahead of time, on weekends or a day off, and freeze for use later. Make double amounts so that there is enough for several meals.

◆ Try to include a salad, fruit, or vegetable with every meal. Have fresh fruit for dessert instead of cake, cookies, or other sweets.

◆ Do not abuse alcohol or drugs to cope with stress. These are not long-term solutions and ultimately will only make you feel worse.

◆ Limit your fast-food meals. When eating fast food, go for pizza some of the time instead of burgers or fried chicken, and don't forget the salad bar.

◆ Take turns packing nutritious lunches and snacks to take to work. This will save you money and discourage you from buying less nutritious lunches at work.

◆ Be sure you and your partner are both clear about the way household and child care responsibilities are to be shared. Remain flexible and make adjustments as necessary to avoid boredom and burnout.

◆ Find some time during the day to do some type of exercise. This could mean an exercise class or a brisk walk around the neighborhood. Getting some type of vigorous exercise three or more times a week is one of the best ways to cope with stress and feel better. If you can't find the time or energy to exercise regularly, remember that any exercise, however infrequently done, is better than none at all.

◆ Try to follow a budget that allows for some freedom to eat out once in a while, go on a vacation, or enjoy some other pleasures.

◆ Practicing the relaxation and visualization exercises you learned in Chapters 4 and 6 can help you cope with stress. Five minutes of relaxation twice a day can be very restoring. And, if you practice these at work, it might give you some energy for the end of the day.

Having a child means that your life is both more routine and more unpredictable at the same time. Children get sick at the most inconvenient times—right before a vacation is to begin, or on an important work day. It will be helpful for you to have one or two people you can call at the last minute to babysit for your child at home.

Try to make some time each week for yourself. It may be difficult to muster the energy to schedule free time, but if you go weeks or months without any, you will become angry and burned out. A burned-out, angry parent can't

take much joy in his or her child. It's in both your interest and the child's for you to have some time for yourself.

Being a working parent is certainly stressful. But to keep things in perspective, you should remember that the amount of time your child is small is very short compared with the entire span of your life. It will take some time after the birth of a child before your life feels normal or manageable again, but it will.

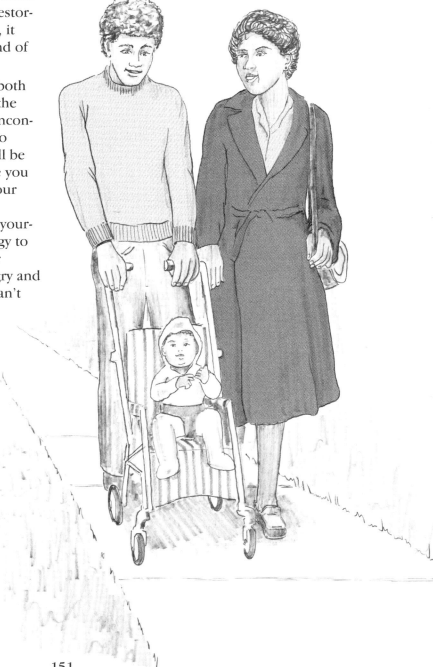

Going Back to Work—Discussion Sheet

Discuss the following questions with your partner and write the answers you agreed on in the spaces provided. You and your partner should then have a good start toward figuring out how to handle child care and home responsibilities when you both work.

There is no answer that is right for everybody. The solutions that work for you and your partner might not work for another couple. Your needs also may change over time. It is important to remain flexible.

1. How much leave will each parent take after the baby is born?

   Mother: _____

   Father: _____

2. Which parent's job is more flexible in terms of allowing for sick leave and not requiring overtime work?

   Mother's: ☐   Father's: ☐

3. Who will take time off from work when the baby is sick or for well-baby checkups?

   Mother: ☐   Father: ☐

4. Who will take the baby to the care giver in the morning?

   Mother: ☐   Father: ☐

   Who will pick up the baby at the end of the day?

   Mother: ☐   Father: ☐

5. How will the responsibilities for doing household chores change for each parent?

   _____

   _____

   _____

   _____

6. What unnecessary household chores can be eliminated?

   _____

   _____

   _____

   _____

7. How can one or both parents adjust their work and social habits to make it easier to share in-home responsibilities (for example, turning down overtime work assignments, limiting out-of-town work trips, limiting social engagements)?

Mother: _____

_____

Father: _____

_____

8. What type of child care does each parent prefer? (See "Child Care Choices," Appendix B.)

Mother: _____

_____

Father: _____

_____

9. Where in your community can you find support? List any groups or community resources you know about that offer support to working parents.

_____

_____

_____

_____

Sex After Baby

Most couples want to know how long they have to wait after the baby is born to have sex. Your health care provider will recommend how long you should wait, but in general, you should wait until your postpartum bleeding stops, your episiotomy or cesarean incisions heal (if you had either), and until you feel like having sex.

The first time you have intercourse after a baby's birth, you may feel some discomfort or pain. A water-soluble lubricant or contraceptive jelly may help. Never use petroleum jelly or any other product that does not dissolve in water. If you had an episiotomy, you may be more comfortable on the top during intercourse.

Couples should be gentle with each other and continue to talk about their needs and desires for physical affection. The best way to ease back into a sexual relationship may be with massage and touching.

Family Planning

You may wonder why it is important to talk about family planning when you are so involved in getting ready to have a baby. What many people do not know is that in the first weeks and months after having a baby a woman may be ovulating even if she isn't having menstrual periods. This is true even if she is breastfeeding. **Breastfeeding is not a form of birth control,** nor are douching, showering after having sex, or having the man withdraw before he ejaculates (comes).

Sometimes a woman going in for her six-week postpartum checkup finds, to her surprise, that she is pregnant again. To avoid an unplanned pregnancy, couples should start using some method of family planning as soon as they resume sexual relations after the baby's birth. Due to changes in the woman's body after childbirth, certain family planning methods might not be effective during the first six weeks postpartum. If you want to avoid getting pregnant during this period, you should abstain from sexual intercourse or use a condom with contraceptive foam, jelly, or cream.

The best method of family planning is the one you will use correctly and consistently. Various methods and a brief description of how they work are given below.

Family Planning Methods

There are many methods of family planning. Your health care provider can give you and your partner detailed information on the methods and tell you if there are medical reasons why any of them would not be a good choice for you.

The most common methods are—

♦ **Birth control pills**—The pills stop the woman's egg from being released from the ovary. They must be taken daily. A woman taking the pills will still have a monthly period. If you are interested in birth control pills, see your health care provider.

♦ **Cervical cap**—The cap covers the woman's cervix and keeps the sperm from entering the uterus. The cap must be used with a spermicide*. If you are interested in the cervical cap, see your health care provider.

♦ **Condom**—The condom covers the man's penis and catches the sperm so that it does not enter the vagina. It is often used with a spermicide* for extra effectiveness. A condom should be used only once and then thrown away. Condoms are available over-the-counter.

♦ **Contraceptive implant**—A contraceptive implant consists of small tubes inserted under the skin of the woman's upper arm. The tubes contain hormones that suppress ovulation. If you are interested in the contraceptive implant, see your health care provider.

♦ **Diaphragm**—The diaphragm covers the woman's cervix and keeps the sperm from entering the uterus. The diaphragm must be used with a spermicide*. If you are interested in the diaphragm, see your health care provider.

---

*Spermicides**—The chemicals in spermicides kill sperm in the vagina. Spermicides are available over-the-counter. A spermicide is a foam, cream, or jelly that is inserted in the woman's vagina.

- **I.U.D. (intrauterine device)**—An I.U.D. is a small plastic device inserted in a woman's uterus. It keeps fertilized eggs from implanting in the uterine wall. If you are interested in an I.U.D., see your health care provider.
- **Natural family planning**—In natural family planning, the woman determines her fertile days by observing changes in her body. She then abstains from intercourse on those days. If you are interested in natural family planning, see your health care provider.
- **Sponge**—The sponge covers the woman's cervix and keeps the sperm from entering the uterus. The sponge contains a spermicide. The sponge is available over-the-counter.
- **Sterilization**—Sterilization involves either the woman or the man being made infertile by surgery. If you are interested in sterilization, see your health care provider.

When you discuss family planning with your health care provider, be sure to ask the following questions about any method you are considering:

- What percentage of women using this method get pregnant?
- If I got pregnant using this method, what would be the risks to my unborn child?
- Would this method affect my ability to have children in the future?
- What are the health risks involved in using this method? Are there any side effects? What are the warning signs that would alert me to seek medical attention?
- What are the advantages and disadvantages of this method?
- Is this method hard or complicated to use?
- How much does it cost?
- How often would I need a checkup if I used this method?
- How would this method affect my breastfeeding my baby?

The Next Step

Now that you have finished Module III, you are ready to begin making decisions about how both your baby and you will be cared for. Following are some of the things you should talk over with the baby's father before the baby is born:

◆ What type of postpartum care would you like for yourself and for your baby? (See Appendix A.)

◆ Will you breastfeed or bottle feed?

◆ If your baby is a boy, do you want to have him circumcised?

◆ Who will be your baby's health care provider?

◆ How will you cope with going back to work?

◆ What child care will you use for your baby?

◆ What will you do about family planning?

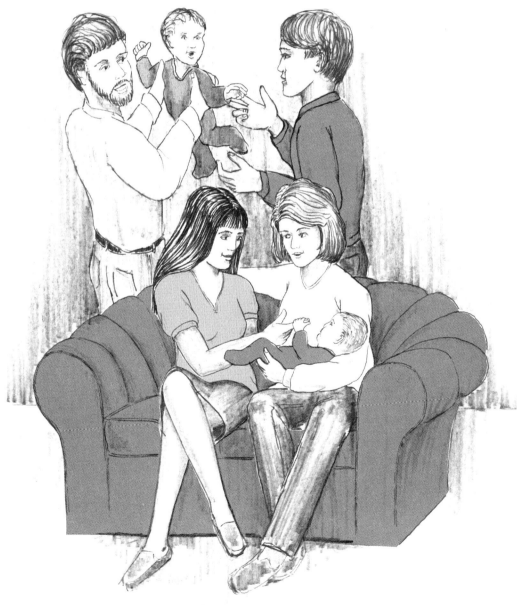

Appendixes

Appendix A: Choices in Childbirth

The checklist below lists some of the choices you may have to make about labor, birth, and the postpartum period. Familiarize yourself with them and discuss them with your health care provider so you will feel confident when the time comes for you to make a choice.

Choice of Health Care Provider
____ OB-GYN
____ Family practitioner
____ Nurse-midwife
____ Midwife

Note: If you have insurance, be sure that the services you choose are covered.

Choice of Birthplace
____ Hospital
____ Birthing center
____ Home
____ Other location

Partner and/or Others Present
____ During labor
____ During birth
____ For all procedures
____ During caesarean
____ During recovery
____ In postpartum room

Early Labor
Perineal Shave
____ None
____ Partial

Enema
____ Routine
____ Only as needed
____ None

Intravenous
____ Routine
____ Only as needed

First Stage of Labor
Takes place in
____ Labor room
____ Birthing room
____ Home

Monitoring the Baby
____ Fetoscope
____ Doptone
____ Electronic fetal monitor
    ____ Internal
    ____ External

Baby Monitored During
____ All of labor
____ Part of labor
____ Only as needed

You Would Like to Be
____ Up and about
____ Confined to room
____ Confined to bed

You Would Like Access to
____ Liquids only
____ Ice chips
____ Nothing by mouth

Membranes
____ Rupture naturally
____ Ruptured by health care provider

Labor Proceeds
____ On its own
____ With artificial stimulation

Medications
____ None
____ As needed
____ Particular medications
_____
_____

Second Stage of Labor
Birth in
____ Delivery room
____ Labor room
____ Birthing room
____ Labor, delivery, recovery, postpartum room (LDRP)
____ Other location

Presence of
____ Other children
____ Other family members

Birthing Position
____ Semisitting
____ Reclining on side
____ Squatting/modified squatting
____ Hands and knees
____ Using stirrups

Lights
____ Bright
____ Dim

Episiotomy
____ Routine
____ Only as needed
____ None

Immediately After Birth

Prophylactic Eye Treatment for Baby
____ Immediately after birth
____ Delayed

Breastfeeding
____ In delivery area
____ In recovery area

Bonding Time With Baby
____ Immediate
____ After baby taken to nursery
____ After baby weighed, measured, and footprinted

Postpartum

Room
____ Private
____ Semiprivate
____ Home

Location of Baby
____ Always stay in mother's room
____ Brought in as necessary
____ Brought in on a predetermined schedule

Method of Feeding
____ Breastfeeding
____ Bottle feeding
____ Combination of both

Length of Stay
____ A few hours
____ One day
____ Several days

Sibling Visitation
____ Limited
____ Unlimited
____ Siblings can have physical contact with baby

Circumcision
____ Yes
____ No

Appendix B: Child Care Choices

Becoming a responsible, loving parent is sure to be one of your greatest challenges. The person or people with whom you leave your child when you are not be with him or her will share this important task with you. You should do everything possible to find quality care for your child.

If you plan to return to work, you should begin shopping around for child care at least several months before you need it. You may find information concerning available child care through your local government, employer, health care provider, childbirth educator, relatives, or neighbors and friends. Child care providers often advertise in local newspapers or family-oriented publications and magazines.

Consider the child's needs. An infant needs individualized care, so at first you may want to consider home care, either in your home or someone else's. As your baby begins to become more social, you may want to consider care in a small group, either in a child care center or a family child care home.

Remember that your child needs responsible care by someone who is calm and affectionate, who likes children, and who accepts your child as he or she is. Your child needs to be surrounded by happy, content adults who enjoy taking care of him or her. Remember, too, that your child's care giver should be well rewarded financially for a job well done.

You must also consider your own needs. Which location would be the best for you, close to home or close to work? Which hours of the day do you need care for your child? Exactly how much can you afford to spend?

References

Whatever type of child care you choose, it is very important that you obtain a list of references and that you check them. When checking the references, you may want to ask some or all of the following questions:
- Was your child happy with the child care?
- Would you choose this care giver again? If not, why?
- What did you like most about this care giver?

- Did you or your child have any problems with the care giver?
- Was the care giver careful about the needs and safety of your child?

Types of Child Care

The three basic types of child care are in-home child care, family child care, and child care centers. Following is a discussion of each type. The discussions include questions you should ask anyone you are considering leaving your child with and suggestions for instructions you should give the care giver you choose.

In-Home Child Care

In-home care means that you pay a person to come into your home to take care of your child. Although this is convenient, it is usually the most expensive option.

To find someone to care for your child in your home, you can read the classified ads in your local paper under "positions wanted" or you can advertise there or in family-oriented publications. In some cities there are referral agencies specifically for child care providers, and they will send candidates to you for consideration. Once you have found several candidates, make arrangements to interview them at your home with your child present. Watch carefully to see how the candidate interacts with your child.

In the interview you may want to ask the candidate the following questions:
- What kind of child care references do you have?
- Have you worked with children before? What were their ages?
- What kinds of things do you like to do with children?
- Do you have children of your own? If so, who is taking care of them?
- Would you take care of my child if he or she is sick?
- Do you know how to use a safety seat correctly?
- Do you smoke? (A candidate who smokes should understand that he or she is not to

smoke around the baby. Consider carefully the health and safety risks of having your child cared for in an environment where smoke, lighted cigarettes, and matches are present. It is best not to hire a smoker for the job.)

- Have you had infant/child CPR or first aid training?
- What other kinds of work experience have you had?
- Why did you leave your last job?
- Are you considering other types of work?
- What are your long-term career goals?

Written Agreement

After you've chosen an in-home care giver, you should put the terms of employment in writing. Include information such as—

- The days and the hours the care giver is to work.
- The amount and terms of payment (including arrangements for sick and vacation time).
- Your wishes concerning visitors, phone calls, television, etc., while the care giver is working in your home.
- Specific policies regarding other tasks you wish the care giver to perform (housework, shopping, preparing meals, etc.). Consider carefully whether having responsibility for other tasks will take the care giver's time and attention away from your child.

Ask the care giver to give you a certificate of health signed by his or her health care provider. This certificate should indicate that the care giver is free from communicable diseases and has a negative TB test result on file. The TB test should have been done in the current calendar year.

Special Instructions

You may wish to leave special instructions, in writing, about the following aspects of your child's care:

- Feeding, such as preparing and handling breast milk or formula, when you expect the child to be hungry, and how the child is best burped.
- Ways to calm your child when he or she is not hungry, but crying, such as favorite positions, special blanket, toys, and books.

- What and how often to feed your child. Include specific don'ts about foods that can cause choking, such as peanuts or hard candy, and foods the child is allergic to.
- Specifics on household safety. Point out all safety features such as fire and smoke alarms, locks, fire escape routes, and fuse box. Also point out any safety concerns you have about your house or apartment. It is a good idea to fix any obvious safety problems, such as short circuits, faulty electrical wiring, and broken glass, before bringing someone into your home to care for your child.
- Use of car safety seat. If, for any reason, your care giver transports your child in an automobile, make sure he or she is able to use the safety seat properly. Take time to show the care giver how to install the seat and let the care giver do it a few times while you watch. Emphasize that the child must always be in the safety seat when traveling in the car.

Emergency Information

Post by the telephone an emergency telephone number list, such as the one in Appendix K. Give the care giver a completed medical care form that authorizes medical care for your child in an emergency. A sample medical authorization form is at the end of this appendix.

Quality of Care

Being concerned about the care your child receives is natural. There are a few things you can do to monitor your child's care:

- Notice your child's disposition when you come home. Does he or she seem happy or sad and fearful? It is normal for the child to be a little upset when you leave but by the time you return, he or she should be happy and comfortable with the care giver.
- Notice if the child is clean.
- Be alert to any injuries your child has, even minor ones. Unlike toddlers who often fall and run into things on their own, babies who are not mobile should not be subject to injuries. If the care giver cannot tell you how your child was injured, or if the child has repeated injuries, you should find a new care giver.

◆ Stop in unexpectedly from time to time to see what is going on. The care giver should be comfortable with this and with your calling to see how your child is doing.

Family Child Care

In family child care, an adult usually takes several children into his or her home during the day. The care giver may or may not have his or her own children to care for. Your child will have other children to play with but only one care giver. Family child care gives a child a home atmosphere and, in most cases, personalized attention. Your county or state may require family child care homes to be licensed. If so, check to be sure that any family child care home you are considering has a valid license. You can receive a copy of the exact regulations on family child care operations in your county or state from the human services agency that governs the licensing.

The best time to check out a family child care home is when care is going on. Make an appointment to interview the care provider. You may want to ask the provider the following questions:

◆ What child care references do you have?
◆ Why did you choose family child care as a profession?
◆ How long have you been providing child care?
◆ How many children do you care for each day and what are their ages?
◆ What do you enjoy doing with the children?
◆ Do you have an enclosed yard for the children to play in or do you take them to the playground?
◆ Will any other person(s) be involved in caring for the children? (If so, ask to meet them.)
◆ Are there any pets in the home? Will they be kept away from the children during the day? (This is important to protect your child from potential injury or in case your child has any allergies to animals.)
◆ What is your policy on sick children?
◆ Are there safety seats and belts for each child you transport in a car?

◆ Have you had infant/child CPR or first aid training?
◆ Are meals and snacks provided to the children? If so, what do they consist of?
◆ Do you smoke? (If so, consider carefully the health and safety risks of having your child cared for in an environment where smoke, lighted cigarettes, and matches are present. It is best not to place your child in a smoker's home.)

Facility Assessment

You should look carefully at the environment itself in a family child care home. Ask for a tour of the areas in which the children are cared for, both inside and outside the house. Make note of the following:

◆ Does the home have a clean and comfortable appearance, but not so clean you'd never know children were present?
◆ Is there enough space indoors and out so all the children have room to move freely and safely?
◆ Are there toys suitable for your child?
◆ Is play equipment safe and in good repair?
◆ Is the outdoor play area fenced and free of litter or debris, including pet waste if the provider has pets?
◆ Is there adequate childproofing in evidence for your child?
◆ Are there safe, clean, quiet places for children to take naps?
◆ Are there separate crib sheets for each child in care?

Written Agreement

It is important to know what policies and procedures are followed by the care giver and to understand and agree with them. If the care giver has no contract of his or her own, you may want to make up your own written agreement and include—

◆ The types of services provided.
◆ The amount and terms of payment, including payment arrangements for sick and vacation time.
◆ The hours and days your child will be in care.
◆ Specific policies, such as care for a sick child and taking field trips.

If the care giver has his or her own contract, review it and add anything that you think is necessary. Ask the care giver to give you a certificate of health signed by his or her health care provider. This certificate should indicate that the care giver is free from communicable diseases and has a negative TB test result on file. The TB test should have been done in the current calendar year.

Special Instructions

You may wish to leave special instructions, in writing, about the following aspects of your child's care:

♦ Feeding, such as preparing and handling breast milk or formula, when you expect the child to be hungry, and how the child is best burped.

♦ Ways to calm your child when he or she is not hungry, but crying, such as favorite positions and special blanket.

♦ What and how often to feed your child. Include specific don'ts about foods that can cause choking, such as peanuts or hard candy, and foods the child is allergic to.

♦ Use of car safety seat. If, for any reason, your care giver transports your child in an automobile, make sure he or she has and is able to properly use a safety seat. Emphasize that the child must always be in the safety seat when traveling in the car.

Emergency Information

Provide the care giver with emergency telephone numbers. You may want to use Appendix K. Give the care giver a completed medical care form that authorizes medical care for your child in an emergency. A sample medical authorization form is at the end of this appendix.

Quality of Care

Being concerned about the care your child receives is natural. There are a few things you can do to monitor your child's care:

♦ Notice your child's disposition when you pick him or her up. Does he or she seem happy or sad and fearful? It is normal for the baby to be a little upset when you leave him or her, but by the time you return, he or she should be happy and comfortable with the care giver.

♦ Notice if the child is clean.

♦ Be alert to any injuries your child has, even minor ones. Unlike toddlers who often fall and run into things on their own, babies who are not mobile should not be subject to injuries. If the care giver cannot tell you how your child was injured, or if the child has repeated injuries, you should find a new care giver.

♦ Stop in unexpectedly from time to time to see what is going on. Your care giver should be comfortable with this and with your calling to see how your child is doing.

Child Care Centers

Child care centers are convenient because they are open from early in the morning until evening. One advantage of center-based care is that it often offers organized preschool activities, sometimes combined with religious or cultural programs. Your child will also have many other children to play with. Unlike some home care situations, all child care centers must meet specific hygiene and safety standards in order to be licensed by the county or state.

If your child goes to a child care center, you might meet other parents whose children attend the center, with whom you can share concerns and possibly develop friendships. Find out if the center encourages communication between parents, as well as whether it encourages parent involvement with the affairs of the center itself.

If you are considering a child care center, visit while the children are there. Make sure the staff-to-children ratio is correct for the age group. The preferred ratio for children younger than two years old is one staff person for every four children. For toddlers, the ratio is one staff person for every six children. You can receive a copy of the exact regulations on child care center operations in your county or state from the human services agency that governs the licensing.

Since children are cared for by several employees at a center, you should get a feel for what type of workplace the center is. Notice whether the workers appear to be enjoying themselves with the children. By interviewing the director of the center, you should be able to get information on the qualifications of the staff and how they are compensated by the center. How well they are paid and the types of benefits they receive will in part determine how high staff morale is at the center. An unhappy worker is most likely not going to have the patience to handle the demands of the children, and child abuse or neglect could be a consequence.

Make an appointment to interview the center director. You may want to ask the director the following questions:

◆ Does the center have an up-to-date license? Was it ever revoked? If so, why?

◆ How much employee turnover is there? (A high rate of employee turnover means that children at the center will have a difficult time forming attachments to their care givers.)

◆ How much are employees paid at the center? Do they get paid sick and vacation leave?

◆ How much experience do the employees have in the child care field?

◆ Have the employees had any early childhood development training?

◆ Is there any continuing education or training provided to employees?

◆ Are the employees certified in infant and child CPR and have they had first aid training?

◆ Does the center have enough safety seats for all the children if they are transported by car?

◆ What types of meals and snacks are served to the children?

◆ What is a typical daily activity schedule for the children?

◆ Do the children play outside for part of each day, weather permitting?

Facility Assessment

Ask for a tour of the center and grounds. Make note of the following:

◆ Does the center have a clean and comfortable appearance, but not so clean you'd never know children were present?

◆ Is there enough space indoors and out so all the children have room to move freely and safely?

◆ Are there enough toys and supplies for all the children in care?

◆ Is play equipment safe and in good repair?

◆ Is the outdoor play area fenced and free of litter or debris?

◆ Is there adequate childproofing in evidence for your child?

◆ Are there safe, clean, quiet places for the children to take naps?

◆ Are there separate crib sheets for each child in care?

Written Agreement

The child care center will have a written contract for you to sign. Be sure to read it carefully and understand all its terms before signing. If you have any special concerns or requests, see that they are included in the agreement. The center should also have its own emergency information and medical care form for you to fill out on your child.

Quality of Care

Being concerned about the care your child receives is natural. There are a few things you can do to monitor your child's care:

◆ Notice your child's disposition when you pick him or her up. Does he or she seem happy or sad and fearful? It is normal for the baby to be a little upset when you leave, but by the time you return he or she should be happy and comfortable with the care giver.

◆ Notice if the child is clean.

◆ Be alert to any injuries your child has, even minor ones. Unlike toddlers who often fall and run into things on their own, babies who are not mobile should not be subject to injuries. If the care giver cannot tell you how your child was injured, or if the child has repeated injuries, you should find a new care giver.

Stop in unexpectedly from time to time to see what is going on. The care givers should be comfortable with this and with your calling to see how your child is doing.

Building a Relationship With Your Care Giver

Whatever type of care you select, it will take time for you, your baby, and the care giver to adjust to the new routine. It is a good idea to stay with your baby for a while the first day or two, or make those first days short ones. Gradually decrease the amount of time you spend at the care giver's. You can expect the child to be upset when you first leave, but he or she should settle down fairly soon.

Trust your instincts about how well things are working out, but also give your child and his care giver a chance to build their own relationship. If, after a reasonable amount of time, you or your child is not happy in the situation, talk it over with your care giver and try to find out why. The quality of this relationship will be very important to you and your baby and is well worth taking time to cultivate and improve.

Emergency Medical Authorization for a Child

Child:

Name _____ Date of birth _____

Phone number _____ Home address _____

Known medical conditions and allergies, if any: _____

Parent(s) or Guardian(s):

Name(s) _____

Phone number(s) _____

Home address(es) _____

Workplace phone numbers(s) _____

Person to contact if parent(s) or guardian(s) cannot be reached:

Name _____ Phone number _____

Address _____

Child's physician or clinic:

Name _____ Phone number _____

Address _____

Health insurance:

Name _____

Address _____

Name of subscriber _____ Identification number(s) _____

I authorize _____ _____
                          (name of care giver)

to obtain immediate medical care for the child named above, and I consent to the hospitalization of, the performance of necessary diagnostic tests upon, the use of surgery on, and/or the administration of drugs to the child if an emergency occurs when I cannot be contacted immediately.

_____   _____
(signature of parent or guardian)   *(date)*

Appendix C: Resources for Overseas Military Personnel and Their Dependents

U.S. military personnel and dependents stationed overseas need specialized information on where to get services and assistance during pregnancy and after their baby is born. Listed below are key resource agencies for Army, Navy, and Air Force personnel who are expecting a baby while stationed outside the United States.

The information provided applies to all services unless otherwise indicated.

I. Obstetrical Care and Childbirth

Contact the patient administration department of the closest military Medical Treatment Facility (MTF) to find out where women receive their care and/or give birth. Information is also available to Navy personnel through Family Services. Possible resources for care include:

A. Local military hospital/clinic
B. Regional military hospital (if the regional hospital is some distance away, the pregnant woman may be sent there to board for several weeks before delivery)
C. Host country physician and/or hospital

II. Birth Registration

The patient administration department of the Medical Treatment Facility has information on birth registration. Procedures may vary according to where you give birth. It is very important that you find out the procedure for this in your area and obtain the necessary documents before the birth of your baby (these documents may include certified birth certificates, marriage certificate, orders, divorce papers) so that birth registration will not be delayed.

If you deliver in a military hospital, you will be issued a "record of birth" document, which you must use to obtain birth registration papers and your baby's passport.

If you deliver in a host country hospital, you will probably be issued a local birth record, which you must use to obtain birth registration and passport.

III. Passport for Infant

The baby's passport must be obtained from the closest U.S. embassy or consulate as soon as the parents receive birth documents. Failure to do so may result in delays if emergency travel out of the country is necessary. Again, check the patient administration department for more information.

IV. Key Resource Agencies

A. Social services, including budget counseling, financial assistance, "loan closet," and emergency food
   1. Army: Army Community Services, social worker services at the hospital, Community Health Nurse
   2. Navy: Family Services, hospital, clinic, Navy Relief
   3. Air Force: Family Services, Personnel, Customer Service, Air Force Aid Society
   4. American Red Cross

B. Food assistance programs available in the United States (WIC, Food Stamps, EFNEP) are not available overseas. The following agencies are available overseas to assist personnel in need of food.
   1. Army: Army Emergency Relief and Community Services Food Locker Program
   2. Navy: Family Advocacy Program (at hospital or clinic), Exceptional Family Member Program, Family Services

C. Counseling/social work services are available at most military Medical Treatment Facilities (MTF)

D. Substance abuse treatment
   1. Army: Community Counseling Centers located on all installations and in military communities.
   2. Navy: Family Services, Family Advocacy Programs (in hospitals and clinics)
   3. Air Force: Mental Health clinic

E. Domestic violence and child abuse/neglect These problems are addressed by the DOD-wide Family Advocacy Program. The Family Advocacy Program provides information,

Appendix C: Resources for Overseas Military Personnel and Their Dependents

incident reporting procedures, and treatment. For service-specific contact agencies, see below.

1. Army: Army Community Services
2. Navy: All clinics and hospitals
3. Air Force: Mental Health clinic

F. Health information
1. Army: Community Health Nurse, expectant parents' classes
2. Navy: hospital, clinic, Family Services
3. Air Force: Health Promotion Coordinator, local hospital or clinic
4. American Red Cross

G. Nutrition counseling
Nutrition counseling is available in hospital facilities and sometimes in clinics. The specific resource agency for each branch of service is listed below.
1. Army: Nutrition Care Division, Community Health Nurse
2. Navy: hospital, clinic, Family Services
3. Air Force: Nutritional Medicine Service

H. Childbearing exercises
Exercise programs for individuals may be available through physical therapists at hospital facilities.

I. Child development/child care services
1. Child care centers provide day care and are available on installations or in military communities. Check for waiting lists for newborns.
2. Certified family day care homes are not available in all areas.

J. Infant equipment and clothing
1. Post/Base Exchange for purchase of equipment and clothing.
2. USAA sells car safety seats to subscribers for wholesale prices.
3. Thrift shops are good sources for furniture, equipment, and clothing.
4. Air Force: Family Services Loan Closet has furniture, equipment, clothing, kitchenware, and other items that can be borrowed on a short-term basis for no charge.
5. Navy: Family Services often has layettes available for mothers in need.

This is your time to take an inner journey to a very special place: the very center of your pregnancy—the womb.

◆

Begin by breathing deeply and rhythmically in through the nose and out either through the nose or slightly parted lips—whichever you prefer.

◆

Become aware of your breathing... and as you do, let your breathing become a little deeper, a little slower, without straining or forcing the breath in any way.

◆

Now, imagine that each breath you take in is a soft, golden, radiant light.

◆

You can think of this light any way you want—as something real: life energy... or as something imaginary: a metaphor for the breath.

◆

Breathe this radiant light right into the center of your being. Let each breath you take in fill you more and more with this soft, golden, radiant light.

◆

And let each breath you let out relax you more and more. Each breath you let out melts tension away more and more.

◆

Now, **mothers**: imagine that you are able to breathe this soft, golden, radiant light directly into your womb.

◆

With each breath in, soft, golden, radiant light fills your womb—the womb that is the center of your pregnancy, the center of all the changes taking place in your body, your emotions, your mind.

◆

Meanwhile, **fathers**: continue to breathe this radiant light into the very center of your being.

◆

And, as you do, imagine that this light is somehow able to connect you, to link you, with your unborn child.

◆

Now, **both mothers and fathers**: imagine that your mind, your consciousness is somehow able to be in the womb with your baby and that you are face to face with your unborn child.

◆

Visualize the baby in any way that feels comfortable to you. You don't have to be concerned with how the baby actually appears at this stage of development. Just picture the baby in whatever way feels right.

◆

Perhaps you want to imagine the baby lying head down, surrounded by a crystal-clear sea of amniotic fluid in his or her own private universe—perfectly comfortable, secure... at peace.

◆

Enjoy being with your unborn child in this unique way for a little while.

◆

And, as you do, if you find your attention wandering or if irrelevant thoughts come into your mind, gently bring your awareness back to your baby by mentally repeating the word "baby" with each breath you let out. Baby... baby... baby.

◆

And let yourself go into an even deeper state of relaxation—body and mind.

◆

Now, allow the love you feel for your baby to well up within you.

◆

(Continued)

And, as you do, you may want to talk with your baby. Tell your baby anything you want: how you are feeling right now... how much you are looking forward to holding him or her in your arms... how much you love him or her... anything you want.

◆

You may even want to ask your baby a question. What do you most need right now?... Where would you like to be born?... What will you most need during the first week after birth?... Any question you wish.

◆

Imagine that your baby can answer you—in words, images, impressions—by painting a picture in your mind's eye.

Don't be surprised if, while doing this exercise, you glimpse the baby's gender or some aspect of the baby's physical characteristics—even the baby's personality. This is perfectly normal.

◆

For now, dwell on the love you feel for your unborn child.

◆

And, as you do this, tell yourself: I am able and willing to give my child everything he or she needs to grow and be healthy....

◆

And when you are ready to return to your everyday waking life, take a few deep breaths, stretch gently and open your eyes.

◆ ◆ ◆

To enhance the bond both parents share with their unborn child, while doing this exercise, focus on the love you and your child share.

To develop confidence in your ability to give birth normally, take a mental tour of the womb. Then express gratitude for the miracle that has already taken place—the creation of your child. Remind yourself that, by the time labor begins, most of the hard work—the creation of the baby—is already over. Of course, there is hard work and pain in labor, but your body has already performed the awesome creative miracle.

To make better birth plans, ask the baby: "Where would you like to be born?" and allow your mind to remain open for a possible "answer."

It is not necessary to believe the child actually answers the question. You can think of the baby as a metaphor for your own inner thoughts.

In "answer" to your question, you may imagine a birth place suffused with peace and love, or you may receive no impression, in which case you will still have opened your mind to consider the birth place from the baby's point of view.

To enhance your intuition ask the baby a question and allow your mind to be open to "receive" an answer. Possible questions are: What do I most need to do to prepare for a safe, positive birth? What will you most need during the first few weeks after birth?

This exercise helps you bypass your logical mind and get in touch with your inner resources. Both are necessary for a rich, full childbirth experience.

Contributed by Carl Jones, author of *Mind Over Labor* and *Visualizations for an Easier Childbirth*.

Appendix E: Labor Telephone List

Fill in the names, addresses, and telephone numbers and post the list by your phone.

Health care provider name _____

Telephone number(s) _____

After-hours telephone number(s) _____

Labor companion name _____

Telephone number(s) _____

Hospital name _____

Telephone number _____

Address _____

_____

Name of person who will care for other children _____

Telephone number(s) _____

Address _____

_____

Emergency medical service (EMS) telephone number _____

Childbirth

Bradley Childbirth Academy
P.O. Box 5224
Sherman Oaks, CA 91413
(818) 788–6662 or (800) 423–2397 or
(800) 42B–IRTH (inside California)
Information about the Bradley method of natural childbirth and Bradley childbirth classes in your area.

American Society of Psychoprophylaxis in Obstetrics (ASPO/Lamaze)
1101 Connecticut Avenue, N.W.
Suite 300
Washington, DC 20036
(800) 368–4404 or (202) 857–1128
Official Lamaze method organization.
Information on local Lamaze groups and childbirth education in general, as well as childbirth education training programs.

International Childbirth Education Association (ICEA)
P.O. Box 20048
Minneapolis, MN 55420
(612) 854–8660
(800) 624–4934 (for book orders only)
One of the largest organizations providing information to the public about pregnancy, birth, and childbirth education. Training programs and referrals to childbirth educators. Large mail-order bookstore. Local affiliations.

Cesarean/Support, Education and Concern (C/SEC)
22 Forest Road
Framingham, MA 01701
(508) 877–8266
Information and support to parents who have had or anticipate a cesarean birth and to those who want to prevent one, as well as parents seeking a vaginal birth after cesarean.
Many local chapters.

Birth and Life Bookstore
P.O. Box 70625
Seattle, WA 98107
(206) 789–4444 or (800) 736–0631
Extensive catalogue of books on every aspect of pregnancy, birth, and parenting. Mail-order service.

Maternity Center Association
48 E. 92nd Street
New York, NY 10128
(212) 369–7300
Information and education about family-centered maternity care.

National Association of Childbearing Centers
3123 Gottschall Road
Perkiomenville, PA 18074
(215) 234–8068
Information on how to select a birth center, as well as a list of free-standing birth centers in the United States. (Cost is $1.)

Breastfeeding

La Leche League International
9616 Minneapolis Avenue
P.O. Box 1209
Franklin Park, IL 60131
(708) 455–7730
Information on breastfeeding and breastfeeding support groups.
Many local chapters.

Parenting

Parents Anonymous
6733 South Sepulveda Boulevard
Suite 270
Los Angeles, CA 90045
(800) 421–0353
Prevention of child abuse. Many local chapters.

Safety

National Safety Council
444 North Michigan Avenue
Chicago, IL 60611–3991
(312) 527–4800 or (800) 621–7619
Infant safety information.

U.S. Consumer Product Safety Commission
Washington, DC 20207
(800) 638–2772
Product safety information.

Death of a Child/Miscarriage

Compassionate Friends
P.O. Box 3696
Oakbrook, IL 60522–3696
(708) 990–0010
Emotional support for parents who have had a miscarriage or lost a child. Over 600 chapters in the United States.
Resource guide and educational material.

National Sudden Infant Death Syndrome (SIDS) Clearinghouse
8201 Greensboro Drive
Suite 600
McLean, VA 22102
(703) 821–8955
Referral service and publications list.

Professional Organizations

American College of Nurse-Midwives (ACNM)
1522 K Street, N.W.
Washington, DC 20005
(202) 289–0171
Lists of certified nurse-midwives and where they attend births.

American College of Obstetricians and Gynecologists (ACOG)
409 12th Street, S.W.
Washington, DC 20024
(202) 638–5577 or (800) 673–8444
Numerous patient education pamphlets.

American Academy of Pediatrics
141 N.W. Point Boulevard
Evanston, IL 60007
Information on infant and child care.

Financial Assistance

Women, Infants and Children Supplemental Food Program (WIC)
Contact your state department of health for a local office.

Department of Social Services
Contact your local department for information about receiving public assistance and medicaid.

Pregnancy and Prenatal Care

Baldwin, Rahima, and Palmarini, Terra. *Pregnant Feelings.* Berkeley: Celestial Arts, 1986.

Blatt, R. *Prenatal Tests: What They Are, Their Benefits and Risks, and How to Decide Whether to Have Them or Not.* New York: Vintage, 1988.

Davis, Elizabeth. *Heart and Hands: A Midwife's Guide to Pregnancy and Birth.* Berkeley: Celestial Arts, 1987.

Eisenberg, Arlene; Murkoff, Heidi E.; and Hathaway, Sandee E., R.N. *What to Expect When You're Expecting.* New York: Workman, 1984.

Kitzinger, Sheila. *Your Baby Your Way: Making Pregnancy Decisions and Birth Plans.* New York: Pantheon, 1987.

Kitzinger, Sheila. *The Complete Book of Pregnancy and Childbirth.* New York: Alfred A. Knopf, Inc., 1989.

Lesko, Wendy, and Lesko, Matthew. *The Maternity Sourcebook.* New York: Warner Books, 1984.

Lubic, Ruth Watson, C.N.M., Ed.D., and Hawes, Gene R. *Childbearing: A Book of Choices.* New York: McGraw-Hill, 1987.

Nilsson, Lennart. *A Child Is Born.* New York: Delacorte Press/Seymour Lawrence, 1990.

Noble, Elizabeth. *Having Twins: A Parent's Guide to Pregnancy, Birth, and Early Childhood.* Boston: Houghton Mifflin, 1980.

Samuels, Mike, M.D., and Samuels, Nancy. *The Well Pregnancy Book.* New York: Summit Books, 1986.

Simkin, Penny. *Pregnancy, Childbirth and the Newborn.* Deephaven, MN: Meadowbrook Press, 1984.

Prenatal Exercise

Noble, Elizabeth. *Essential Exercises for the Childbearing Year.* Boston: Houghton Mifflin, 1988.

Olkin, Silvia K. *Positive Pregnancy Fitness: A Guide to a More Comfortable Pregnancy and Easier Birth Through Exercise and Relaxation.* New York: Avery Publishing, 1987.

Nutrition

Brody, Jane. *Jane Brody's Nutrition Book.* New York: Bantam, 1987.

Eisenberg, Arlene; Murkoff, Heidi E.; and Hathaway, Sandee E., R.N. *What to Eat When You're Expecting.* New York: Workman, 1986.

(Information on nutrition during pregnancy and lactation is also included in many of the books listed under Pregnancy and Prenatal Care and Breastfeeding.)

Childbirth

Baldwin, Rahima. *Special Delivery.* Berkeley: Celestial Arts, 1987.

Inch, Sally. *Birthrights: What Every Parent Should Know About Childbirth in Hospitals.* New York: Pantheon, 1985.

Jones, Carl. *Alternative Birth: A Complete Guide.* Los Angeles: Jeremy Tarcher, Inc., 1991.

Jones, Carl. *After the Baby Is Born.* New York: Henry Holt & Co., 1990.

Kitzinger, Sheila. *The Experience of Childbirth.* New York: Penguin, 1984.

Kitzinger, Sheila. *Giving Birth: How It Really Feels.* New York: Farrar, Straus, & Giroux, 1989.

Lieberman, Adrienne B. *Easing Labor Pain.* Garden City, NY: Doubleday, 1987.

McCartney, Marion, C.N.M., and Van der Meer, Antonia. *The Midwife's Pregnancy & Childbirth Book.* New York: Henry Holt & Co., 1990.

McCutcheon-Rosegg, Susan, and Rosegg, Peter. *Natural Childbirth, the Bradley Way.* New York: E.P. Dutton, 1984.

Noble, Elizabeth. *Childbirth With Insight.* Boston: Houghton Mifflin, 1983.

Todd, Linda. *Labor and Birth: A Guide for You.* Minneapolis: ICEA, 1981.

Cesarean Birth and Vaginal Birth After Cesarean

Hausknecht, Richard, and Heilman, Joan Rattner. *Having a Caesarean Baby.* New York: Plume, 1991.

Jones, Carl. *The Expectant Parent's Guide to Preventing Cesarean.* Westport, CN: Greenwood, 1991.

Mitchell, Kathleen, and Nelson, Marty, R.N. *The Cesarean Birth Experience.* New York: Kampmann Books, 1985.

Richards, Lynn Baptisti. *The Vaginal Birth After Cesarean (VBAC) Experience: Birth Stories by Parents and Professionals.* South Hadley, MA: Bergin and Garvey, 1987.

Rosen, Mortimer, and Thomas, Lillian. *The Cesarean Myth: Choosing the Best Way to Have Your Baby.* New York: Viking Press, 1989.

Relaxation and Visualization

Benson, Herbert, M.D., and Klipper, Miriam Z. *The Relaxation Response.* New York: Avon, 1976.

Jones, Carl. *Mind Over Labor.* New York: Penguin, 1988.

Jones, Carl. *Visualizations for an Easier Childbirth.* Deephaven, MN: Meadowbrook Press, 1988.

Mitchell, Laura. *Simple Relaxation: The Mitchell Method for Easing Tension.* North Pomfret, VT: David and Charles, 1988.

Samuels, Mike, M.D., and Samuels, Nancy. *Seeing With the Mind's Eye: The History, Techniques and Uses of Visualization.* New York: Random Books, 1975.

For Fathers and Labor Support Partners

Cain, Kathy. *Partners in Birth.* New York: Warner Books, 1990.

Greenberg, Martin. *The Birth of a Father.* New York: Continuum, 1985.

Jones, Carl. *Birth Partner's Handbook.* Deephaven, MN: Meadowbrook Press, 1989.

Jones, Carl. *Sharing Birth: A Father's Guide to Giving Support During Labor.* Westport, CN: Greenwood, 1989.

Simkin, Penny. *The Birth Partner: Everything You Need to Know to Help a Woman Through Childbirth.* Boston: Harvard Common Press, 1989.

For Children

Anderson, Sandra Van Dam, R.N., and Simkin, Penny R.P.T. *Birth—Through Children's Eyes.* Seattle: Pennypress, 1981.

Malecki, M. *Mom and Dad and I Are Having A Baby!* Seattle: Pennypress, 1982.

Premature Birth and Pregnancy Loss

Borg, Susan, and Lasker, Judith. *When Pregnancy Fails.* Toronto, New York: Bantam Books, 1989.

Friedman, Rochelle, and Gradstein, Bonnie. *Surviving Pregnancy Loss.* Boston: Little, Brown, & Co., 1982.

Harrison, Helen, and Kositsky, Ann. *The Premature Baby Book: A Parent's Guide to Coping and Caring in the First Years.* New York: St. Martin's Press, 1983.

Breastfeeding

Dana, Nancy, and Price, Anne. *The Working Woman's Guide to Breastfeeding.* Deephaven, MN: Meadowbrook Press, 1987.

Eiger, Marvin S., M.D., and Olds, Sally Wendkos. *The Complete Book of Breastfeeding.* New York: Workman, 1987.

Kitzinger, Sheila. *Breastfeeding Your Baby.* New York: Alfred A. Knopf, 1989.

La Leche League International. *The Womanly Art of Breastfeeding.* New York: Plume, 1987.

Pryor, Karen. *Nursing Your Baby.* New York: Harper & Row, 1973.

Parenting

Brazelton, T. Berry, M.D. *Working and Caring.* Reading, MA: Addison-Wesley, 1985.

Brazelton, T. Berry, M.D. *Families: Crisis and Caring.* New York: Ballantine, 1989.

Jaffe, Sandra S., and Viertel, Jack. *Becoming Parents: Preparing for the Emotional Changes of First-Time Parenthood.* New York: Atheneum, 1979.

Olds, Sally Wendkos. *The Working Parents' Survival Guide.* Rocklin, CA: Prima Publishing and Communications, 1989.

Richmond, Gary. *Successful Single Parenting.* Eugene, OR: Harvest House Publishing, 1990.

Spock, Benjamin, M.D. *Dr. Spock on Parenting.* New York: Pocket Books, 1989.

Weiss, Robert S. *Going It Alone: The Family Life and Social Situation of the Single Parent.* New York: Basic Books, 1981.

Infant Care and Development

Baldwin, Rahima. *You Are Your Child's First Teacher.* Berkeley: Celestial Arts, 1989.

Better Homes and Gardens. *Better Homes and Gardens New Baby Book.* New York: Bantam, 1986.

Brazelton, T. Berry, M.D. *Infants and Mothers.* New York: Doubleday, 1983.

Briggs, Dorothy C. *Your Child's Self-Esteem.* New York: Dolphin Books, 1975.

Leach, Penelope. *The First Six Months: Getting Together With Your Baby.* New York: Alfred A. Knopf, 1987.

Leach, Penelope. *Your Baby and Child From Birth to Age Five.* New York: Alfred A. Knopf, 1987.

McClure, Vimala Schneider. *Infant Massage: A Handbook for Loving Parents.* New York: Bantam, 1989.

Samuels, Mike, M.D., and Samuels, Nancy. *The Well Baby Book.* New York: Summit Books, 1979.

Spock, Benjamin, M.D., and Rothenberg, Michael B., M.D. *Dr. Spock's Baby and Child Care.* New York: Pocket Books, 1985.

Stoppard, Miriam, M.D. *The First Weeks of Life.* New York: Ballantine, 1989.

Family Planning

Winstein, Merryl. *Your Fertility Signals: Using Them to Achieve or Avoid Pregnancy, Naturally.* St. Louis: Smooth Stone Press, 1990.

Appendix H: Immunization Record

Date	Age	Immunization	Provider
_____	2 months	Diphtheria-pertussis-tetanus (DPT) vaccine and polio vaccine, Hemophilus type b conjugate vaccine (Hib vaccine)*	_____
_____	4 months	DPT vaccine and polio vaccine, Hib vaccine	_____
_____	6 months	DPT vaccine, Hib vaccine	_____
_____	12 months	TB (tuberculosis) test	_____
_____	15 months	Measles, mumps, rubella (MMR) vaccine, Hib vaccine	_____
_____	16–24 months	DPT vaccine, polio vaccine	_____
_____	4–6 years	DPT vaccine, polio vaccine	_____
_____	11–12 years	MMR vaccine	_____
_____	12–16 years	Tetanus-diphtheria (TD) vaccine	_____
_____	Every 10 years thereafter	TD vaccine	_____

*Hib vaccine protects infants and children from meningitis, pneumonia, epiglottitis (a severe form of croup), and other serious infections.

Appendix I: Myths and Facts About Safety Seats

Myth	Fact
A child is safer in a mother's arms.	The forces of impact are too great for an adult to hold a child. A 10-pound baby would weigh the equivalent of 300 pounds in a 30-mph crash. Moreover, on point of impact, adults often crush the child between themselves and the dashboard or door.
Safety seats are inconvenient to use. They take too much time to fuss with.	Some models are more convenient than others. Note, too, that it takes more time to dress and feed a child properly than to strap him or her into one of these seats. Buckling a child in a safety seat is another way of ensuring the child's health.
A household baby carrier can be used as a safety seat.	Household carriers cannot withstand the stresses of a crash. They are flimsy, fragile, and susceptible to breakage in an accident. The sharp edges are an additional danger.
Children don't need to be buckled up because they're small, light, and resilient.	Young children are **more** likely to be thrown about inside the vehicle or out through a window during a crash because they are small and have such large, heavy heads in proportion to their bodies. Most life-threatening injuries suffered by children in motor vehicle crashes are head injuries.
Safety seats aren't important.	Safety seats reduce the chance of death from a crash by 71 percent and serious injury by 67 percent. There are laws requiring the use of safety seats or belts for children.
Safety seats are too expensive.	Loaner seat programs offer seats for a specified period of time for a minimal fee and deposit. Moreover, the cost of a safety seat is negligible when compared to the value of a child's life.
Children can just be placed in the safety seat. They don't have to be buckled in.	The safety seat must be properly fastened to the vehicle with a lap belt first. The belt must be looped through the correct places in order for it to work. In addition, some seats require a tether strap to anchor the seat in the car; a seat that requires a tether must be anchored. Finally, the child must be fastened in the seat by the snugly fastened harness and/or protective shield.
Safety seats themselves can cause injuries.	If the seat is not properly fastened to the car and the child is not properly buckled in the seat, both the seat and child can be thrown about in the car. If the child and seat are properly fastened, such injuries are rare and would be far less severe than what an unprotected child would encounter.

Myth	Fact
Safety seats don't have to be used if the child sits in the back seat.	Unbuckled rear seat occupants, whether adults or children, can pose a danger to front seat passengers. In many crashes, the rear seat occupants are either hurled into the front seat or out the back window.
When there are no safety belts, a safety seat doesn't have to be used.	Safety belts can be purchased from and installed by a local car dealer or van conversion shop. Never allow a child to ride unprotected.
Children don't like safety seats. They feel confined and complain too much.	If children ride buckled from birth, they will be less likely to object later. Children who get used to riding buckled in are more comfortable in safety seats and are better behaved as passengers. These seats are designed specifically to cradle and support small bodies. Unrestrained children, on the other hand, are subject to a lot of bumping and sliding around during the stopping and cornering of normal driving. In addition, there is greater potential for falling off seats or out doors and for causing great distraction for the driver.

Adapted with permission from the *1991 Family Shopping Guide to Car Seats.* Copyright 1991. American Academy of Pediatrics.

Buckling your children up shows you care about their safety.

More children in the US are killed and crippled in car crashes than from any other cause of injury. Therefore, it is now the law in every state that infants and children must ride buckled up in car seats or seat belts.

When used correctly, car seats provide excellent protection in most crashes. Car seats keep children from being slammed into the windshield or dashboard, thrown against other people, or flung out of the car in even a low-speed collision. They also keep children in their places, so that you, the driver, can pay attention to the road.

Choosing a Car Seat

- The "best" car seat is one that fits your child's size and weight, fits in your car, and is used correctly on every ride.
- Check the label to make sure the seat meets current federal safety standards.
- Try the seat in your car to make sure it fits properly.
- Understand that low- and high-priced models generally provide equal crash protection. Higher prices usually mean convenience features, which make the seat easier to use correctly.
- Wide and "T"-shaped shields are equally effective.
- Look for a seat that is easy to use, with straps that are simple to adjust and a seat belt route through which your car's belt can be fastened easily.
- If you **must** get a used seat, look at the label on the seat to make sure it was made after January 1, 1981. Those made earlier do not meet the same strict crash standards. Be sure to get instructions and all parts for any used seat.

Basics of Car Seat Use

- Always use a car seat, starting with your baby's first ride home from the hospital. Help your child form a lifelong habit of buckling up.
- Follow the manufacturer's instructions. Using a car seat the wrong way means your child may not be protected. (Keep the instructions handy.)
- Check your owner's manual for special directions on using the vehicle seat belts with a car seat.
- Remember that the harness and/or shield holds the child in the car seat and the vehicle seat belt holds the seat in the car. Unless **both** are attached snugly, the car seat may not prevent injury.
- If the lap part of a lap/shoulder seat belt doesn't stay tight around the car seat, check the car seat instructions about using a metal locking clip.
- Never use a seat that has been in a crash.

Using Car Seats Correctly _____

Infant Seats (birth to 20 pounds)

Advantage: Small and portable. Gives best fit for newborns.
Disadvantage: Must be replaced by a convertible seat when outgrown.

- Install an infant car seat facing the back of the car, so that the seat supports the baby's body and head during a crash.
- Never use an infant car seat facing forward.
- The seat may rest against the dashboard or against the back of the front seat when used in the rear seat.
- Use the infant car seat until your child reaches 20 pounds and can sit up well alone.
- Route the seat belt through the right place on the car seat and pull it tight.
- Adjust the harness snugly over the shoulders and between the legs.
- Keep the shoulder straps in the slots at or just **below** the baby's shoulders.
- Use a plastic harness clip at armpit level to keep the shoulder straps in place, if provided.
- To keep a newborn from slouching, pad the sides of the seat and the space between the crotch and the harness with rolled up diapers or receiving blankets.
- If an infant's head flops forward, tilt the seat back a little by wedging padding under the base of the seat, just enough so the head stays upright.
- Do not use a household "infant carrier" as a car seat.
- **Premature infants** should be watched in a car seat before discharge from hospital to see if the semi-reclined position adds to possible breathing problems. If the physician recommends, a car bed may be used for a short period so the baby can lie flat.

Infant Car Seat
– facing rearward –

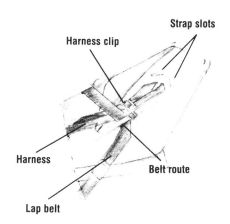

Convertible Seats (birth to 40 pounds)

Advantage: Fits child from birth to 40 pounds (about age 4).
Disadvantage: Bulky. Less portable than an infant car seat.

- Use a convertible seat facing the **rear** for babies up to 20 pounds (see "Infant Seats" for usage tips).
- For children over 20 pounds who can sit up well alone, use the convertible seat facing forward.
- Use a convertible seat until the child reaches about 40 pounds.
- Keep the harness snug, and readjust it as your child grows or changes outer clothing. Use a plastic harness clip at armpit level to hold shoulder straps in place, if provided.
- Thread the shoulder straps through the harness slots at or just **above** the child's shoulders, in the forward-facing position.
- Make sure the seat belt is routed through the car seat correctly in both forward and rear-facing positions (there are usually two different routes); pull the belt tight.
- If you have an older seat that requires a top tether strap when facing forward, be sure to install it. Newer models do not need tethers, although use of an optional tether gives extra protection.

Convertible Car Seat
– facing forward –

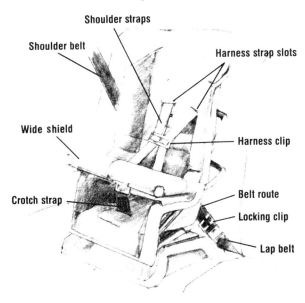

Shoulder straps

Shoulder belt

Harness strap slots

Wide shield

Harness clip

Crotch strap

Belt route

Locking clip

Lap belt

Booster Seats (for children who have outgrown convertible seats)

Belt-Positioning Booster Seats (30 to 65 pounds)

Advantages: Uses vehicle shoulder belt to protect upper body and head. Preferred to shield booster when a lap/shoulder belt is available.
Disadvantage: Cannot be used in seating positions with lap belts only.

- The booster base will raise a child up so lap and shoulder belts fit properly.
- It can be used for children who outgrow their convertible seats below 40 pounds.
- Some models have a separate shield that is added for use when only a lap belt is available (preferrably over 40 pounds).

Shield Booster Seats (40 to 65 pounds)

Advantage: Provides better protection than a lap belt alone.
Disadvantage: Gives less protection than a convertible seat or belt-positioning booster.

- This type is suitable only when a child has reached about 40 pounds, even if labeled for use at a lower weight limit.
- Small shield boosters provide more protection than lap belts alone if the lap belt does not fit very tight and low on the hips or if the child slouches so it rides up dangerously high onto the tummy.
- Never use a booster seat with a lap belt alone unless the booster has a shield.

Booster Car Seat
– facing forward –

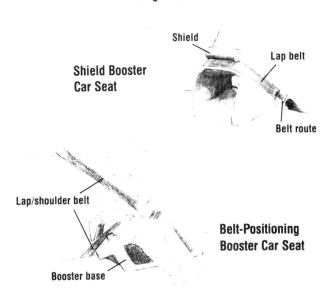

Shield Booster
Car Seat

Shield

Lap belt

Belt route

Lap/shoulder belt

Booster base

**Belt-Positioning
Booster Car Seat**

1991 Shopping Guide to Car Seats

All products listed meet current Federal Motor Vehicle Safety Standard 213

Manufacturer/Name	Harness Type	Harness Adjustment	Special Notes	Price Range
Infant Seats				
Century 560, *565*	Straps only	One-step	Tilt-indicator, fits in shopping cart.	$25-35
Century 580, *590*	Straps only	580 - Manual 590 - One-step	Tilt-indicator; 590 - separate base stays in car; can also be used in car without base.	$45-65
Cosco Dream Ride	Straps only	One-step	To 17 lbs; use flat as car bed, or semi-reclined, rear-facing.	$59-69
Cosco TLC	Straps only	Manual		$29-35
Evenflo Dyn-O-Mite	Straps only	Manual	Shoulder belt wraps around front of seat.	$29-34
Evenflo Joy Ride	Straps only	Manual	Shoulder belt wraps around front of seat; "Joyride Convertible" model is for infants only.	$36-60
Evenflo Travel Tandem	Straps only	Manual	Separate base stays belted in car; seat can be used in second car without base; locks in shopping cart.	$62-79
Fisher-Price Infant Car Seat	Straps/T-shield	Manual	No locking clip; leveling line; locks in shopping cart.	$50
Kolcraft Rock 'N Ride	Straps only	Manual	No harness height adjustment.	$29-50
Convertible Seats				
Babyhood Mfg. Baby Sitter	Straps only	Manual	Previously called "Wonda Chair."	$89
Century 1000 STE	Straps only	One-step	2 crotch strap positions.	$50-60
Century 2000 STE	Straps/T-shield	One-step	2 crotch strap positions.	$55-70
Century 3000 STE, *3500 STE Premier*	Straps/wide shield	One-step	2 crotch strap positions.	$80-90
Century 5000 STE, *5500 STE Premier*	Straps/wide shield	One-step	2 crotch strap positions; multi-position shield; back pads for infant support.	$90-120
Cosco 5-Pt	Straps only	One-step	Back pads for infant support.	$55-59
Cosco Luxury 5-Pt	Straps only	One-step	Back pads for infant support.	$69-89
Cosco Comfort Ride	Straps/wide shield	One-step	Back pads for infant support.	$75-89
Cosco Soft Shield	Straps/T-shield	One-step	Back pads for infant support.	$79
Cosco Autotrac	Straps/T-shield	Automatic	Back pads for infant support.	$99
Evenflo One-Step	Straps/wide shield	Manual		$56-90
Evenflo Champion	Straps/wide shield	One-step	Smaller, lighter than other Evenflo models.	$76-90
Evenflo Seven Year Car Seat	Straps/wide shield	One-step	Converts to booster (see Evenflo Booster).	$110-130
Evenflo Ultara I, II, V	Straps/shield; Straps only (V)	One-step	Wide shield (I); T-shield (II); back pads for infant support.	$90-126
Fisher-Price Car Seat	Straps/T-shield	Automatic	No locking clip provided.	$78
Gerry Guardian	Straps/T-shield	Automatic	Harness locks on impact.	$55-85
Kolcraft Auto-Mate	Straps/T-shield	One-step	New name for "Dial-A-Fit."	$45-75
Kolcraft Traveler 700	Straps/wide shield	One-step		$45-75
Nissan Infant/Child Safety Seat*	Straps/T-shield		Not for aircraft use.	$100
Playskool Carseat (by Kolcraft)	Straps/wide shield	One-step	Inflatable head support for infant.	$70-90
Renolux GT 2000	Straps only	Manual		$60-80
Renolux GT 5000	Straps only	Manual	High headrest; swivel base.	$100-130
Renolux GT 7000	Straps only	Manual	High headrest; remote control recline feature.	$180-200
Harnesses				
Little Cargo Auto Safety Vest (25-40 lbs)	Straps only	Manual	Padded shoulder, hip and crotch straps; auto lap belt attached through padded stress plate.	$40
E-Z-On Vest (several sizes)	Straps only	Manual	Tether strap must be installed in vehicle.	$62

Booster Seats	Belt Position	Special Notes	Price Range
Century Commander*	Wrap-around	Not for aircraft use.	$20-30
Century CR-3*	Wrap-around	**Belt-positioning booster for lap/shoulder belt use;** shield to add for lap belt use; not for aircraft use.	$30-40
Cosco Explorer	Wrap-around	2 seat heights.	$25-29
Evenflo Booster Car Seat	Wrap-around or through base	Split shield open in middle; belt through base for short child; internal crotch strap.	$46-55
Evenflo Sightseer	Wrap-around		$29-34
Gerry DoubleGuard	Wrap-around; through base with lap belt	**Belt-positioning booster for lap/shoulder belt use;** shield to add for lap belt use.	$45-60
Kolcraft Tot Rider Quik Step	Wrap-around	Crotch post; shield pivots down on for access to seat.	$19-35

*Seat not certified for use in aircraft.   (New models in italics.)

Appendix K: Instructions for Emergency Telephone Calls

Emergency Telephone Numbers

EMS _____ Fire _____ Police _____

Poison Control Center _____

Other Important Telephone Numbers

Name of child's health care provider _____

Office number _____

Mother's name _____ Work number _____

Father's name _____ Work number _____

Neighbor's name _____ Home number _____

Name and address of medical facility with 24-hour emergency cardiac care

_____

Telephone number _____

Information for Emergency Call (Be prepared to give this information to the EMS dispatcher.)

1. Exact location of the emergency

   Street address _____

   If you live in a multifamily building give the:

   Name of building _____

   Floor _____ Apartment or room number _____

   City or town _____

   Directions (cross streets, landmarks, etc.) _____

   _____

2. Telephone number from which the call is being made

3. Your name

4. What happened (baby fell, choked on food, won't wake up, etc.)

5. Condition of the baby (baby choking, not breathing, unconscious, etc.)

6. Help (first aid) being given

Note: Do not hang up first. Let the EMS dispatcher hang up first.

American Red Cross First Aid:
When an Infant Is Choking
(Birth to One Year)

For a Conscious Infant

1 Is Infant Choking?

2 Shout, "Help!"

Call for help if infant:
- Cannot cough, cry, or breathe.
- Is coughing weakly.
- Is making high-pitched noises.

3 Phone EMS for Help
- Send someone to call an ambulance.

4 Turn Infant Facedown
- Support infant's head and neck.
- Turn infant facedown on your forearm.

5 Give 4 Backblows
- Lower your forearm onto thigh.
- Give 4 backblows forcefully between infant's shoulder blades with heel of hand.

6 Turn Infant Onto Back
- Support back of infant's head and neck.
- Turn infant onto back.

7 Give 4 Chest Thrusts
- Place middle and index fingers on breastbone.
- Quickly compress breastbone ½ to 1 inch with each thrust.

Repeat steps 5, 6, and 7 until object is coughed up or infant starts to cough, cry, or breathe.

If infant becomes unconscious, place infant on a firm, flat surface.

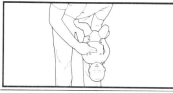

8 Look for Object in Infant's Throat
- Grasp tongue and lower jaw and lift jaw.
- If you can see object in throat, try to remove it with a finger sweep.

To Do a Finger Sweep
- Slide finger down inside of cheek to base of tongue.
- Sweep object out.

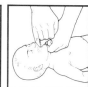

9 Open Airway
- Tilt head gently back and lift chin.

10 Give 2 Slow Breaths
- Keep head tilted.
- Seal your lips tight around infant's nose and mouth.
- Give 2 slow breaths for 1 to 1½ seconds each.

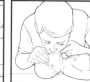

11 Give 4 Back Blows

12 Give 4 Chest Thrusts

Repeat steps 8, 9, 10, 11, and 12 until airway is cleared or ambulance arrives.

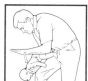
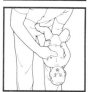

Local Emergency (EMS) Telephone Number:

Everyone should learn how to perform the above steps and how to give rescue breathing and CPR. Call your local American Red Cross chapter (chapter telephone number) for information on these techniques and other first aid courses.

American
Red Cross

American Red Cross First Aid:

When an Infant Stops Breathing

(Birth to One Year)

1 **Does Infant Respond?**
- Tap or gently shake infant's shoulder.
- Shout, "Are you OK?"

2 **Shout, "Help!"**
- Call people who can phone for help.

3 **Roll Infant Onto Back**
- Roll infant toward you slowly.
- Support back of head and neck as you roll infant.

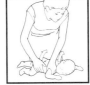

4 **Open Airway**
- Tilt head gently back and lift chin.

5 **Check for Breathing**
- Look, listen, and feel for breathing for 3 to 5 seconds.

6 **Give 2 Slow Breaths**
- Keep head tilted back.
- Seal your lips tight around infant's mouth and nose.
- Give 2 slow breaths for 1 to 1½ seconds each.

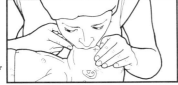

7 **Check for Pulse in Upper Arm**
- Feel for pulse for 5 to 10 seconds.

8 **Phone EMS for Help**
- Send someone to call an ambulance.

9 **Begin Rescue Breathing**
- Keep head tilted back.
- Lift chin.
- Give 1 slow breath every 3 seconds.
- Look, listen, and feel for breathing between breaths.

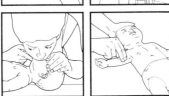

10 **Recheck Pulse Every Minute**
- Keep head tilted back.
- Feel for pulse for 5 to 10 seconds.
- If infant has pulse but is not breathing, continue rescue breathing. If no pulse, begin CPR.

Local Emergency (EMS) Telephone Number: _____

Everyone should learn how to perform the steps above, how to give first aid for choking, and CPR. Call your local American Red Cross chapter _____ (chapter telephone number) for information on these techniques and other first aid courses.

American Red Cross

Glossary

Glossary

Acquired immune deficiency syndrome (AIDS)—The collection of illnesses resulting from infection with the human immunodeficiency virus (HIV).

Afterbirth—Placenta and membranes expelled after the birth of a child.

After-pains—Uterine pains experienced after childbirth as the uterus begins to contract and return to normal size.

Alveoli—Milk glands in the breasts which, when stimulated by the hormone prolactin, produce a flow of milk.

Amniotic fluid—Bag of waters. The fluid surrounding the fetus in the uterus.

Anesthetic—Medication that produces partial or complete insensibility to pain.

Areola—The dark-colored skin surrounding the nipple.

Bag of waters—*See* Amniotic fluid.

Birth canal—Vagina. The vagina receives the penis during intercourse and is the path through which the baby passes during delivery.

Braxton Hicks contractions—Contractions of the uterus that occur throughout pregnancy, but that might not be noticed until the ninth month. Also called "rehearsal contractions."

Breech presentation—The position of a baby who is bottom down rather than head down in the uterus.

Cervix—The neck, or opening, of the uterus.

Cesarean birth—The surgical delivery of the baby through a cut in the abdominal and uterine walls.

Circumcision—A surgical procedure in which the foreskin is cut from the penis, usually performed on an infant soon after delivery.

Colostrum—The first milk from the mother's breasts after the birth of a child.

Conception—Fertilization. The union of the male sperm and the female ovum (egg).

Contraction—The regular tightening of the uterine muscles as they work to dilate the cervix in labor and to press the baby down the birth canal.

Couvade syndrome—Physical symptoms experienced by a man that mimic those of the pregnant woman. They may include nausea, food cravings, back pain, and weight gain.

Effacement and dilatation—The thinning (effacement) and opening (dilatation) of the cervix during labor.

Egg—Ovum. The female reproductive cell produced by the ovary.

Electronic fetal monitoring—The continuous monitoring of the fetal heart by an instrument placed on the mother's abdomen over the area of the fetal heart or by an electrode inserted through the cervix and clipped to the baby's scalp.

Embryo—The term used for the developing baby in the uterus from about the 10th day after fertilization until about the 12th week of pregnancy.

Engagement—Dropping or lightening. Engagement occurs when the baby has settled deep in the pelvic cavity. This often happens in the last month of pregnancy.

Engorgement—The overcongestion of the breasts with milk. May occur if there is too lengthy a time between feedings.

Episiotomy—Surgery performed on the opening of the vagina to enlarge the area and prevent tearing as the newborn emerges.

False labor—Braxton Hicks contractions that come so strongly and regularly that they are mistaken for labor contractions.

Fertilization—*See* Conception.

Fetus—The term used for the developing baby in the uterus from the 12th week of pregnancy until delivery.

Fontanels—The "soft" membrane areas in the skull of the newborn that have not yet turned to bone.

Fundus—The upper part of the uterus.

Health care provider—The term used for doctor, nurse, physician's assistant, nurse midwife or midwife, and nurse practitioner.

Hemorrhoids—Swelling of the blood vessels near the anus.

HIV—*See* Acquired immune deficiency syndrome (AIDS).

Hormone—A chemical substance originating in an organ, gland, or in certain cells of an organ, which is carried by the blood to stimulate various organs to action.

Immunization—Medications given to protect against disease.

Induction—The process of artificially starting labor and keeping it going.

Jaundice—Yellowing of the white areas of the eyes or skin caused by an excessive amount of bilirubin in the blood.

Kegel exercise—Voluntary contraction of the pelvic floor muscles.

Labor—The action of the uterus contracting and the cervix opening to bring about the birth of a baby.

Lactation—The secretion of milk from a woman's breasts.

Lanugo—The fine soft body hair of the fetus.

Let-down reflex—The flow of milk into the nipple from the milk ducts.

Ligament—A fibrous tissue binding and connecting bones.

Lochia—Postnatal vaginal discharge.

Mastitis—An infection of the breast.

Meconium—A dark-green mucus in the intestine of the full-term fetus. It is passed during the first days after birth. The presence of meconium in the amniotic fluid before delivery is usually taken as a sign of fetal distress.

Milia—Small, white blemishes that appear on the face of a newborn.

Molding—The shaping of the bones of the baby's skull as it passes through the birth canal.

Morning sickness—Nausea and vomiting sometimes occurring during the early months of pregnancy.

Mucous plug—Mucus at the tip of the cervix that acts as a barrier into the uterus to guard against infection.

Nutrient—A nourishing food that helps to build and repair body tissue, provide heat and energy, and regulate the body processes; generally classified as proteins, carbohydrates, fats, minerals, and vitamins.

Ovum—*See* Egg.

Oxytocin—A hormone secreted by the pituitary gland that stimulates uterine contractions and the release of milk from the breast. Pitocin is the man-made equivalent of oxytocin and is sometimes given to induce or speed up labor.

Pelvic floor—The muscular structure that supports the bladder and the uterus.

Pelvis—The bones forming a girdle around the hips.

Perineum—The region between the anus and vagina.

Pica—A craving to eat nonfood items such as hair, clay, or sand.

Pitocin—*See* Oxytocin.

Placenta—A spongy mass that grows on the wall of the uterus to which the fetus is attached by the umbilical cord and through which the fetus receives its nourishment and gets rid of waste products.

Glossary

Placenta previa—A potentially life-threatening condition in which the placenta lies over the cervix.

Postpartum—The term used to describe conditions and events that take place after childbirth. It usually applies to six to eight weeks after delivery.

Premature infant—An infant born before the 37th week of gestation or weighing less than 5-1/2 pounds at birth.

Prenatal—The term used to describe something that exists or occurs before birth.

Presentation—The position of the fetus in the uterus before and during labor.

Quickening—The first noticeable movements of the fetus.

Sexually transmitted diseases (STDs)—Diseases transmitted through sexual contact.

Sperm—The male reproductive cell, produced by the testicles.

Station—A measurement indicating where the presenting part of the baby is in relation to the middle of the pelvis.

Trimester—In pregnancy, a period of three months' duration. Pregnancy is divided into three trimesters.

Umbilical cord—The cord that connects the baby to the placenta. It contains veins and arteries through which the baby is nourished and through which waste products are carried away.

Uterus—Womb. The hollow organ in which the fertile egg is embedded and where it develops into the embryo and then the fetus.

Vagina—*See* Birth canal.

Vernix—A white, creamy substance that covers the baby while he or she is in the uterus.

Womb—*See* Uterus.

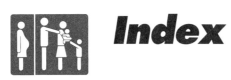 **Index**

Index

Index

Notes

Notes

Notes

Notes

Notes

Notes

MISSION OF THE AMERICAN RED CROSS

The American Red Cross, a humanitarian organization led by volunteers and guided by its Congressional Charter and the Fundamental Principles of the International Red Cross Movement, will provide relief to victims of disaster and help people prevent, prepare for, and respond to emergencies.

ABOUT THE AMERICAN RED CROSS

To support the mission of the American Red Cross, nearly 1.5 million paid and volunteer staff serve in some 1,600 chapters and blood centers throughout the United States and its territories and on military installations around the world. Supported by the resources of a national organization, they form the largest volunteer service and educational force in the nation. They help people prevent, prepare for, and cope with emergencies, whether those emergencies involve blood, disasters, tissue transplants, social services, or health and safety.

The American Red Cross provides consistent, reliable education and training in injury and illness prevention and emergency care, providing training to nearly 16 million people each year in first aid, CPR, swimming, water safety, and HIV/AIDS education.

All of these essential services are made possible by the voluntary services, blood and tissue donations, and financial support of the American people.

FUNDAMENTAL PRINCIPLES OF THE INTERNATIONAL RED CROSS AND RED CRESCENT MOVEMENT

HUMANITY

IMPARTIALITY

NEUTRALITY

INDEPENDENCE

VOLUNTARY SERVICE

UNITY

UNIVERSALITY